Springer Series on
Health Care and Society

Steven Jonas, M.D., *Series Editor*

Advisory Board:

Steven Jonas is Associate Professor, Department of
Community Medicine, at the State University of New
York, Stony Brook, and in 1977–78, Visiting
Professor, Program in Health Facilities Planning
and Design, Columbia University School of
Architecture. He received his B.A. from Columbia
College, his M.D. from Harvard Medical School, and
his M.P.H. from the Yale School of Medicine.
Dr. Jonas, a Fellow of the American Public Health
Association, the American College of Preventive
Medicine, and the New York Academy of
Medicine, is currently President of the Association of
Teachers of Preventive Medicine. He is the author
of *Medical Education in the United States* (1978),
editor of *Health Care Delivery in the United States*
(Springer, 1977), and Chief Editor of the new
Springer Series, "Health Care and Society."

Quality Control of Ambulatory Care

A Task for Health Departments

STEVEN JONAS, M.D.

SPRINGER PUBLISHING COMPANY

NEW YORK

Springer Publishing Company, Inc.
200 Park Avenue South
New York, N.Y. 10003

77 78 79 80 81/ 10 9 8 7 6 5 4 3 2 1

Designed by Patrick Vitacco

Library of Congress Cataloging in Publication Data

Jonas, Steven.
    Quality control of ambulatory care.

    (Health care & society)
    Includes index.
    Bibliography: p.
    1. Ambulatory medical care—New York (State)—
Quality control. 2. Poor—Medical care—New York
(State). 3. New York (City)—Hospitals—Outpatient
services. 4. Clinics—New York (State)—Suffolk Co.
I. Title. II. Series. [DNLM: 1. Quality control.
2. Ambulatory care. WX205 J75q]
RA981.N7J66   362.1   77–24502
ISBN 0–8261–2240–X
ISBN 0–8261–2241–8 pbk.

To my parents,
Professor Emeritus Harold J. Jonas
and Mrs. Florence K. Jonas, M.A.

Contents

Foreword

Ambulatory care is the most prevalent form of health service delivery in the United States. It is the commonest scene of encounter between the patient and the health professional, ranging from visits to the solo practitioner's office to the hospital-based outpatient department or the freestanding group practice. In any kind of national health insurance plan, ambulatory care is bound to play a major role because as utilization of services increases with greater access, it will become essential to protect the more expensive forms of service—the hospital and nursing home beds—from overuse and to shift the burden of service to ambulatory care whenever possible.

While the setting for ambulatory care deserves study in its own right, it has been more often neglected than not. This monograph appropriately raises the question of the impact of national health insurance on ambulatory care and examines examples of government-funded ambulatory care programs in New York State as prototypes of how the government can provide subsidy and at the same time control expense and quality.

The findings are somewhat disheartening. The New York State Health Department had for many years paid little attention to the quality of ambulatory care services in hospitals and clinics although it had the responsibility to do so. Nor did the subsidized Ambulatory Care Program in New York City and in Suffolk County, the two areas chosen for examination, receive adequate attention from governmental authorities. The New York City Health Department began an exemplary monitoring program of Ghetto Medicine clinics in New York City, but, unfortunately, this effort has not been continued. The difficulties described in this volume of implementing ambulatory programs in Suffolk County, a largely rural area, are particularly striking.

Clearly, much is still to be learned about the best form of ambulatory care should this become the major vehicle for national health insurance. A contract method may provide the best set of controls but may also be quite inflexible, or patients may cling to the services of their familiar solo practitioner even when enrolled in a health maintenance organization. If so, how will the government and the patient be assured of quality? Many physicians will welcome institutional or group practice, but many will resist. If an adequate reporting system is established, it is not inconceivable that individual practitioners could be monitored for quality. Encounter forms can provide information to be fed into a central computer. Out of this, physician and patient profiles can be constructed that will give vast amounts of data that could be used on a sampling or spot-check basis to determine if reasonable amounts of care of high quality are being delivered. In fact, Medicare and Medicaid have already prepared physician performance profiles. Special incentives can offer rewards for development of more efficient team practice using allied health professionals. Second opinion programs for surgery and major diagnostic procedures can help enforce standards.

The Joint Commission on Accreditation of Hospitals is now gearing up to extend its review procedures to ambulatory settings. Professional Standards Review Organizations are also developing criteria for peer review of ambulatory care. By the time a national health insurance plan is enacted, it is very likely that adequate monitoring methods will be in place to attempt to control the costs and assure the quality of office encounters between patients and physicians. Whether all these efforts will be successful is yet to be determined.

Meanwhile, this monograph provides a clear look at some of the problems and points the way to possible solutions. It is a distinct step forward in bringing order to the examination of ambulatory care, in many ways the most important segment of the health care delivery system, and as such, it is a major contribution. The author is to be congratulated for his diligence and perspicacity in defining a major area for research and attention in the future.

New York, 1977

GEORGE G. READER, M.D.
Livingston Farrand Professor
and Chairman
Department of Public Health
Cornell University Medical College

Preface

In anticipation of the advent of some form of national health insurance in the United States within the foreseeable future, the New York Metropolitan Regional Medical Program established in 1974 a "Task Force on the Impact of National Health Insurance on the State of New York." The Task Force carried on a number of different activities. Among them was the commissioning of a series of special studies and position papers both on general health care system problems and on particular health care systems problems and programs in New York State. These studies were intended to help answer the Task Force's major question: "What do we do when national health insurance comes?"

This monograph is one of the special studies in revised form. The original study was commissioned by the first staff director of the Task Force, Professor Irving Lewis, to examine the enforcement of quality standards for ambulatory care in hospitals by the New York State Department of Health under Article 28 of the State Public Health Laws and by the New York City Department of Health under the so-called Ghetto Medicine program, renamed the Ambulatory Care Program. Early in the study it was determined that such a focus would be too narrow, and the study was broadened to include general histories of Article 28 and Ghetto Medicine and some general evaluations of both programs beyond simply their effects on ambulatory care quality.

The original report is entitled *Organized Ambulatory Services and the Enforcement of Health Care Quality Standards in New York State: It Doesn't Matter How Many Teeth You Have if You Can't Close Your Mouth.* It was delivered to the Task Force on June 27, 1975. An abridged version of the original report will appear in the final report of the Task Force. This monograph includes most of the text from the original study, plus some additional analytical material and a relatively brief selection from the appendixes which accompanied the original report. Those appendixes, listed herein in Appendix 1, contained over 300 pages.

I was the study director for the project. In collecting and considering the meaning of the data, I was ably assisted by several persons. Stephen Rosenberg, M.D., M.P.H., assistant professor at the Columbia University School of Public Health and Administrative Medicine, was the senior consultant in New York City. He had a major responsibility for collecting and analyzing material on the New York City Department of Health Ambulatory Care Program. He was assisted by Ms. Christine Gunston, a student at the school. Nancy Barhydt, R.N., M.A., assistant professor, Department of Community Medicine, Albany Medical College, was the senior consultant in Albany, New York. She had a major responsibility for collecting and analyzing material on Article 28. She was very ably and energetically assisted by Bruce La Flamme, a student in the School of Social Welfare, State University of New York at Albany.

Ms. Virginia Neary, a student in the School of Social Welfare, Health Sciences Center, State University of New York at Stony Brook, carried out the study of the Ghetto Medicine program in Suffolk County. Chapter 7 is condensed from her original report. I was greatly assisted at Stony Brook by Charles Andrews and Daniel Ricciardi, undergraduate students. I acknowledge with many thanks the participation of all these individuals, without whom the study could not have been undertaken and completed, with special thanks, of course, to my principal coworkers, Dr. Rosenberg, Prof. Barhydt, and Ms. Neary.

The original study was supported, of course, by the Task Force, and I am grateful to them for providing me and my colleagues the opportunity to carry out a most stimulating piece of research.

The report on which the bulk of this monograph is based is used with the kind permission of the New York Metropolitan Regional Medical Program, Jesse Aronson, M.D., director, and of the Task Force, Marvin Lieberman, Ph.D., staff director. The views and positions expressed in this book do not necessarily reflect those of either the Task Force or the New York Metropolitan Regional Medical Program.

Portions of chapters 2 and 3, "Hospital Ambulatory Services" and "Health Care Quality Measurement and Control" are taken from chapters 6 and 13 in *Health Care Delivery in the United States,* which I edited, published by Springer Publishing Company, New York, 1977. I wrote chapter 13 and coauthored chapter 6 with Barbara Rimer, M.P.H. The material is used with the permission of Ms. Rimer and Springer Publishing Company.

The preparation of this monograph was made possible in part by the generous support of the Josiah Macy, Jr., Foundation, New York, New York, and of my father, Harold J. Jonas. I acknowledge their help with many thanks.

The typing of the original report and this monograph was done principally by Eugenia DiGirolamo, Eleanor Lindwall, and Jeffrey Elhai. I thank them for their invaluable help.

Finally, the reader will note that the original report was based almost entirely on material gathered in a series of personal interviews. This is due in large part to the fact that there is a paucity of both primary and secondary printed sources, both published and unpublished, concerning the programs studied. Therefore, we are most grateful to those persons whom we interviewed (see app. 2). Without their assistance, of course, neither the original report nor this monograph could have been written.

1

Introduction

The Basis of the Study

It is likely that a national health insurance program (Jonas, 1974, 1977b; House of Representatives, 1974; Eilers, 1971; Weinerman, 1971; Bodenheimer, 1972) will be enacted in the United States in the next five years, with a good chance that enactment will take place within the next two years. Large sums of money which are now spent by people for health services, either directly out of pocket or through private health insurance plans, will be spent through a legally mandated health insurance program, operated either by government or by the private insurance industry under government regulation. As is well known, there are many serious concerns with the structure of the health care system in the United States and with the overall character of the services it delivers (Committee on the Costs of Medical Care, 1970; Battistella and Southby, 1968; Jonas, 1977a; R. Roemer, Kramer, Frink, & M. Roemer, 1975; Silver, 1976). Two of the many important problem areas are regulation and quality control on the one hand, and the provision of ambulatory care (non-inpatient care) in organized settings (other than in private practice) on the other.

One useful technique for improving knowledge and understanding of any problem area is historical analysis of previous experience which is similar in at least certain aspects to the predicted future experience. The Task Force on the Impact of National Health Insurance on the State of New York, for which this study was done, used this approach in a number of different areas. A discussion paper by Herbert Lukashok and Eric Ploen examined the issue of ambulatory care in voluntary hospitals in the city of New York

1

(1974). Among the issues which they considered is the problem of improving the organization of ambulatory services provided by voluntary hospitals. In this regard, they stated:

> Pressure on the hospitals for the restructuring of ambulatory serv- ices will probably not come specifically from the National Health Insurance legislation or subsequent regulations. Rather govern- mental stimulus and influence on a Federal level will likely be forthcoming from those programs designed to provide underpin- ning to the health care system in preparation for National Health Insurance. Two such broad programs are already here—the PSRO's [Professional Standards Review Organizations] and the HMO's [Health Maintenance Organizations]. Most important in this connection will be legislation creating a nation-wide network of organizations to be known as Health Systems Agencies. . . .
>
> However, in New York on both the State and local levels there is additional machinery already available that could be useful in accomplishing this objective.
>
> The same article 28 of the New York State Public Health Laws which requires the approval as to public need to the State Health Commissioner for the construction of new or additional hospital beds, authorizes him to "inquire into the operations of hospitals and to conduct periodic inspections of facilities with re- spect to the fitness and adequacy of the premises . . . and stand- ards of medical care." (Sec. 2803–1)
>
> Further, the law also states that "the State Hospital Review and Planning Council shall adopt rules and regulations . . . to effec- tuate the purposes of this article including (a) the establishment of requirements for uniform state-wide system of reports and audits relating to quality of medical and physical care pro- vided. . . . (Sec. 2803–2) Within the State Hospital Code man- dated by article 28, there already exists provision relating to the quality of care in ambulatory services. . . .
>
> On a city level the standards for ambulatory services devel- oped by the [City] Health Department in order for hospitals to receive Ghetto Medicine subsidy represent a most creative attempt to tie money to program development and improvement. . . .
>
> There are obviously serious difficulties in supervision and en- forcement of these codes and standards. The point to be empha- sized, however, is that there already exist in New York precedents and framework to move hospitals to adopt programs deemed desirable, necessary, and in the public interest. (pp. 8–9)

Although this analysis was written in reference to voluntary hospitals, a similar one can be applied to local government hospitals as well, and indeed to other types of organized settings from which ambulatory care is provided: Health Maintenance Organizations of various sorts, neighborhood health centers, local health department centers, and the like. In raising the questions with which the original report was concerned, Irving Lewis, then Staff Director of the Task Force, stated the following on February 21, 1975, in a personal letter to me:

> If national health insurance is enacted, we can anticipate that it will substantially enlarge the benefits for outpatient care and will thus create great pressures—not easily quantified—upon our existing capacity for delivering ambulatory care. A major part of this capacity is the voluntary hospital. It is important, therefore, to inquire into what can be done at the state and local level to influence or direct the voluntary hospital to provide the desired ambulatory service.
>
> In order to proceed with this inquiry, we formulate the thesis that precedents in the city and the state have already been established for setting of standards, monitoring the quality of care, and mandating performance or effectiveness. These precedents exist in Article 28 requirements and the Ghetto Medicine Act.

In relation to these concerns, the following specific questions were asked by Professor Lewis:

1. What was the intent of the law (Article 28) and how was it expressed in law, Hospital Code, and regulations?
2. What was supposed to happen under these programs, what did happen, and, if the answers differed, why did they?
3. How did the Department of Health respond to the enactment of Article 28 insofar as ambulatory care is concerned? What is the history of the development of the appropriate portions of the Hospital Code, e.g., were they merely lifted from elsewhere or do they represent intentionally planned developments? What were the sources for standards?
4. In practice, what is the effective power of the Health Department, state or local, regardless of what the regulations state? What sanctions exist, and what experience has there been in using them?

5. What inspection schedules exist, with what reality and what resources? What questions are covered in inspections?
6. On Ghetto Medicine specifically, we need a funding history as well as the legislative history and in general whether, in the last analysis, the program had made any real difference—not in funding hospital deficits, but in assuring the availability and access of services and their restructuring. Thus, we ask what demands were placed on hospitals, what was the hospitals' response, and how was the response monitored? Did changes occur in their ambulatory services, were they for the better and, if not, why not?
7. What are the dynamics of changing the Hospital Code? What is the process of amendment, who has the power to amend, is it relatively easy or difficult to amend, etc.?

Our original study set out to answer these questions. This monograph considers three different governmental approaches to the problems of ambulatory care delivery in organized settings. The approach under Article 28 and related provisions of the Public Health Laws of the State of New York is that of standard-setting with enforcement through inspection and regulation. Under the so-called Ghetto Medicine law of New York State, two other approaches have been tried. One is subsidy of efforts of local-government departments of health to provide general medical services through health department centers and other means. The other is the contract method which has been used by the New York City Health Department to provide money to help voluntary hospitals in the city operate their inhospital ambulatory services, called the Ambulatory Care Program (ACP).

In the final part of this chapter, we report on our methodology. Chapters 2 and 3 consider some of the general issues in ambulatory care and health care quality measurement and control. Chapter 4 covers the New York State Health Department and Article 28 of the Public Health Laws of the State. Chapter 5 considers the historical development of Ghetto Medicine and New York City's Ambulatory Care Program. Chapter 6 reports on the ACP as it operates currently. Chapter 7 looks at Ghetto Medicine in Suffolk County. In chapter 8 conclusions are drawn from the data, and the implications of the study for national health insurance are discussed.

Methodology

INFORMATION GATHERING

The study on which this monograph is based was carried out during a three-month period, March–May 1975. Because of the limitations of time and resources, the study relied primarily on the personal interview method of information gathering. Interviews were carried out with (1) one or more persons in various directorial positions at nine of the ten leading Ghetto Medicine hospitals in New York City (as ranked by the United Hospital Fund, see chap. 6), and persons in directorial positions in Suffolk County Ghetto Medicine Programs; (2) community leaders in New York City and Suffolk County; (3) leading officials in the New York State, New York City, and Suffolk County Health Departments. A complete list of persons interviewed is provided in Appendix 2. We also reviewed the very limited published literature on Article 28 and Ghetto Medicine, the applicable laws and codes, and certain unpublished materials which were made available to us. These sources are referred to in the text, and certain of the most important ones are reproduced in the appendixes.

ANALYSIS OF RESEARCH TECHNIQUES

In this study, we used the first stage of the scientific method—description. Existing information, experiences, points of view, and analyses concerning the problem were gathered, and a descriptive picture was assembled. No attempts at statistical analysis or experimentation were made. Although this approach has its limitations, for most problem areas it is necessary to do a descriptive study first so that requirements for more rigorous study can be clearly delineated. We used the descriptive approach only, not proceeding to either retrospective or prospective study, primarily because of limitations of time and resources.

Several points should be made about our use of the descriptive method. In interviewing, all interviewers used the open-ended method, without a structured questionnaire. We did not want interviewees to be strait-jacketed. We wanted to be flexible so that the discussions could concentrate on those areas in which interviewees were most interested and in which they could be most helpful. Also, we did not want the different interviews to be repetitive, since we were not intending to carry out statistical operations on interview results. We conducted a fairly large number of interviews, so that, even without a structured questionnaire, we feel certain that, with perhaps a few exceptions, we have our facts straight. With the free format, then, we feel that we sacrificed nothing in assembling the historical pictures which we wanted, while at the same time we gained a great deal by obtaining a wide variety of viewpoints and perspectives from a panel of interviewees representing a broad cross section of points of participation in relevant parts of the health care delivery system.

Although the major methodological technique was the interview, we also reviewed published papers, public documents, and some relevant unpublished material to reinforce, add to, and fill gaps in the information gained by interviews. Certain pieces of quantitative data are found in these sources, but we present them only as support for our descriptive approach.

In terms of the quality of the descriptive data itself, several caveats must be entered. Interviews with representatives of hospitals concerning both Article 28 and the ACP were carried out in New York City, while Article 28 is a state law. Although we have included in our report some general material on Article 28 implementation, we were concerned principally with the relationship of Article 28 to organized ambulatory care. The major portion of hospital ambulatory care other than emergency room services in New York State is carried out in hospitals in New York City. A complete picture would indeed require a consideration of the experience in the other major cities in the state and in a sample of nonurban hospitals, but we feel that, on the basis of our results, such a picture would differ little if at all from that which we derived from an analysis of the New York City experience.

Our analysis of the implementation of Ghetto Medicine outside of New York City is limited to only one county's program. However, the program outside of New York City is limited in its extent, and Suffolk County appears to be prototypical for those counties which have made an effort to do anything.

In sum, we have carried out a descriptive study of the defined problem area, and, within the boundaries of that technique, have produced results which we feel are a valid representation of reality. We recognize the limitations of that approach, and among our recommendations are several quantitative analyses which could answer questions which descriptive techniques cannot. Nevertheless, it will be seen that certain policy recommendations can justifiably be made simply on the basis of information gathered by the descriptive technique.

References

Battistella, R., & Southby, R. McK. F. Crisis in American medicine. *Lancet*, 1968, *1*, 581.

Bodenheimer, T. The hoax of national health insurance. *American Journal of Public Health*, 1972, *62*, 1324.

Committee on the Costs of Medical Care. Medical care for the American people. Chicago, 1932. Reprinted U.S. Dept. of Health, Education, and Welfare, Washington, D.C., 1970.

Eilers, R. D. National health insurance: What kind and how much? *New England Journal of Medicine*, 1971, *284*, 881, 945.

House of Representatives, Committee on Way and Means. *National health insurance resource book*. Washington, D.C.: U.S. Government Printing Office, 1974.

Jonas, S. Issues in national health insurance in the United States of America. *Lancet*, July 20, 1974, p. 143.

Jonas, S. Introduction. Chap. 1 in S. Jonas (Ed.), *Health care delivery in the United States*. New York: Springer Publishing Co., 1977.(a)

Jonas, S. National health insurance. Chap. 15 in S. Jonas (Ed.), *Health care delivery in the United States*. New York: Springer Publishing Co., 1977.(b)

Lewis, I. Personal communication to S. Jonas, Feb. 21, 1975.

Lukashok, H., & Ploen, E. Ambulatory care in voluntary hospitals. Task Force on the Impact of National Health Insurance. New York Metropolitan Regional Medical Program. Process, Dec. 9, 1974.

Roemer, R., Kramer, C., Frink, J., & Roemer, M. *Planning urban health services*. New York: Springer Publishing Co., 1975.

Silver, G. *A Spy in the house of medicine*. Germantown, Md.: Aspen Systems Corp., 1976.

Weinerman, E. R. Organization and quality of service. *Yale Journal of Biology and Medicine*, 1971, *44*, 133.

2

Hospital Ambulatory Services

Introduction

Ambulatory care is commonly defined by exclusion. It is a personal or combined health care service given to a person who is not a patient in bed in a health care institution. A *personal* health service is defined as a preventive, treatment, or rehabilitative service given to an individual patient, benefitting principally that patient alone, such as setting a fractured ankle. A *community* health service is one given to a population rather than to individuals, such as the provision of a pure water supply. A *combined* health service is one given to an individual, which service has both personal and community aspects, such as immunization against measles. Thus the term *ambulatory care* covers all health services other than personal and combined services given to institutionalized patients and community health services.

Since there are about three times as many visits to physicians on an ambulatory basis annually as there are hospital days of care (Danchik, 1975, Table B; American Hospital Association, 1976, Table 1), it can be concluded that the majority of physician-patient contacts in the United States take place on an ambulatory basis. As White points out, "the vast bulk of care is provided by physicians in ambulatory settings. Only 10 percent of the people [seen] are admitted to a hospital . . ." (White, 1973, p. 29).

About half the material in this chapter comes from chapter 6, "Ambulatory Care," by Steven Jonas and Barbara Rimer, in *Health Care Delivery in the United States*, edited by Steven Jonas (copyright © 1977 by Springer Publishing Company, Inc., N.Y.). It is used with the permission of the publisher and Miss Rimer. Most of the balance of the material comes from the original report.

There are two major categories of ambulatory care. One, by far and away the largest, is care given by private physicians in solo, partnership, or private group practice on a fee-for-service basis. The other can be called ambulatory care in organized settings. An organized setting here is taken to mean a locus of medical practice with an identity which is independent of that of the particular individual physician(s) working in it. This category includes hospital-based ambulatory services (primarily clinics and emergency care), emergency medical services systems, health department clinics, prepaid group practices, Foundations for Medical Care, Health Maintenance Organizations, neighborhood health centers, organized home care, community mental health centers, industrial health services, school health services, and prison health services. In this chapter, we limit our discussion to hospital-based ambulatory care.

HISTORICAL DEVELOPMENT OF HOSPITAL AMBULATORY SERVICES

The institutional center of the American health care system is the hospital. For a variety of historical reasons (Freymann, 1974, chap. 3), the majority of American hospitals focus the bulk of their efforts and activities on patients who are acutely ill and confined to bed —the inpatients. Hospitals, however, have also had to deal with a variety of other types of patients. Among them are those presenting themselves for care who do not require admission to a bed, immediately at least—the outpatients. In terms of the relative emphasis most hospitals give to the two groups of patients, the names could not have been better chosen.

Voluntary hospitals. There are two historical streams of development of organized ambulatory care in the United States, both of which are related to the care of persons not able to pay for their own medical care (Freymann, sec. 2). Beginning in the eighteenth century, the voluntary, charitable sector of the health care system built hospitals which, on their inpatient services, devoted themselves in part to caring for people not able to pay for their own care. (In fact, there were not too many paying patients, because hospitals could not do very much for their patients in any case.) However, all patients admitted to voluntary hospitals had to have "curable" diseases—that is, limited, acute ones—whether or not they could pay. In the nineteenth century, voluntary hospitals began to develop outpatient services as well, almost entirely for the poor. At the same time, separate organized ambulatory care institutions—dispensaries—were developed by independent charitable organizations, or by voluntary hospitals uninterested in establishing ambulatory services within their own walls (Rosenberg, 1974, p. 32). They were the distant forebears of the contemporary neighborhood health centers, in function at least. In that century, almost all voluntary dispensaries were absorbed into voluntary hospitals. There were local government dispensaries as well. Dispensaries were an important factor in urban medical care at one time (Rosenberg, p. 33). In 1900, there were about 100 of them in the United States. In New York City alone in that year, dispensaries provided over 800,000 visits. However, they were poorly staffed, poorly financed, and viewed with displeasure by private practitioners, who saw them as competing for patients. They were considered as distinctly second-class institutions. Most of them had disappeared by the 1920s (Rosenberg, p. 49).

By the end of the nineteenth century, clinic service was part of the functions of most hospitals serving the poor in urban areas (Freymann, chap. 3, 4). Until the late nineteenth century, hospitals were relatively uncommon in the United States. In 1875, there were fewer than 200 of them (Stevens, 1971, p. 52). A building boom then took place, and by 1909 there were 4,359 hospitals, with a bed capacity of 421,000.

By 1916, 495 hospitals had clinics, in many cases serving an educational as well as a charitable function (M. Roemer, 1975, p. 38). However, the clinics certainly shared the second-class status of the dispensaries. When, for example, a clinic was built onto the archetypical nineteenth-century voluntary hospital, the Johns Hopkins in Baltimore, it was added at the back (Freymann, 1974, p. 56). This typified the approach. As Freymann says (p. 200): "It was and still is an appendix tacked on the periphery of the bed-filled tower that soaks up the pride and wealth of the community. The ambulatory services huddle at the nether end of the pecking order. . . ."

Local government hospitals. The second stream of development for organized ambulatory services is the local government hospital sector (Freymann, sec. 2). Local government hospitals developed from poor houses and have always had the means-test principle as a basic element of their institutional being. They have also tended to embody, with a few recent exceptions, the poor-law principle of "less eligibility." Local government hospitals have always had a larger role in ambulatory services than voluntary hospitals, but their ambulatory services have suffered for two reasons: the institutions have been treated as second-class, and the physicians who staff them by and large have been trained in and often still work in a voluntary sector which itself treats hospital ambulatory services as an "obligation" and as useful for teaching and research. Furthermore, the original requirement that voluntary hospitals had for caring only for "curable" patients has remained an important psychological force (Freymann, p. 29).

This has been reinforced in modern times by the "interesting case syndrome" which has developed in both kinds of institutions when they are involved in teaching medical students or house staff. For reasons which we shall not go into here, "interesting" has come to be synonymous with "rare" or at least "relatively infrequent." Of course, there is nothing intrinsically more "interesting" about a rare disease than there is about a common disease. It is simply a matter of teaching, role-modeling, and socialization of the student provider. This type of mind set has not led to the development of hospital ambulatory services which are especially beneficial to the bulk of patients using them, who, it happens, have relatively common rather than relatively uncommon health problems.

The Basic Two: Clinics and Emergency Rooms

Outpatients can present themselves to a hospital for either immediate treatment for an acute and often serious illness or injury, or care for a more routine matter requiring medical attention but not necessarily immediately. Very often, the services required by the latter type of patient are very similar to those needed by patients who attend private practitioners' offices. Although there are some exceptions, the former group of patients goes to the emergency unit, while the latter group goes to the clinics. The increasing confusion in the minds of hospital staffs and administrations and of patients themselves trying to unravel the complexities of the health care system has resulted in increasing difficulties in sorting out the differences in role and function of the two divisions and in deciding who should go where for what.

Historically, it apparently has been easier for hospitals to make a determination that emergency services should be provided rather than that clinic services should be. About 85 percent of community hospitals[1] in the United States (4,882 in 1975) have emergency units (American Hospital Association, 1976, Table 12A). The original intended function of emergency units was to take care of people acutely ill or injured, particularly with life-threatening or potentially life-threatening problems, requiring immediate attention with personnel and/or equipment not found in private practitioners' offices, and potentially requiring early hospitalization. Most hospitals have found it desirable or necessary to provide such services.

On the other hand, historically the hospitals which have paid the most attention to clinic services have been those located in areas in which patients could not or would not attend private practitioners' offices for more routine care, usually for economic reasons (M. Roemer, 1971) and/or which have teaching programs. Only about one-quarter of community hospitals (1,421 in 1975) have clinics (American Hospital Association, 1976, Table 12A). It is probably not coincidental that emergency outpatient services, particularly for critically ill patients, are not among those services that private physicians can easily provide in their own offices, whereas the type of service provided in clinics can usually be given by private physicians, economic considerations aside.

In considering problems of hospital ambulatory services, it should be kept in mind that they are not of one type nor are they found only in one category of hospital. Most of the literature on hospital ambulatory care in the United States deals with the situation in university and other teaching hospitals. Thus, we are probably being presented with a distorted picture of what is really going on. Excluding Veterans' Administration Hospitals (about which we also know little), approximately 65 percent of emergency department visits and 40 percent of clinic visits take place in non-medical–school-affiliated hospitals (American Hospital Association

---

1. The American Hospital Association defines a community hospital as a "short-term, general, and other special hospital."

1976, derived from Tables 3 and 8). However, medical-school-affiliated hospitals do set a great deal of the hierarchical tone in the United States, and thus it is useful to look at what goes on in them.

Hospital Clinics

Functions. Clinics today have their historical role of care for the poor, although little "free" care remains. At best, patients have some third-party coverage, and at worst are faced with a means–test-related sliding-fee scale. Then, despite their second-class status, clinics do have a teaching function, for medical students and house staff. Finally, many clinical researchers have found the outpatient clinics to be a useful place to work. However, the research function, and to a considerable extent, the teaching function, have led to organizational problems which have resulted in confusion and conflict.

Types. The best way of organizing outpatient clinics to provide opportunities for teaching and research, especially in view of the way contemporary medical education is structured, is to have a large number of disease–, organ–, or organ–system-specific clinics (Freymann, 1974, p. 255). The typical contemporary teaching hospital has three groups of clinics: medical, surgical, and other. The medical clinic group may or may not have a "general medical clinic" which approximates the function of the general internist. It always has an array of specialty clinics: cardiology, neurology, dermatology, allergy, gastroenterology, and so on. Patients may stay in one or more specialty clinics for long periods of time, particularly in the typical situation in which the general medical clinic is small or nonexistent; and specialty clinics admit patients directly without referral from a general clinic. In the surgical group, there is an array of specialty clinics as well. Since surgical care is usually more episodic than is medical care, patients are not as likely to remain in these clinics for long periods of time. The third group includes pediatrics and the pediatric subspecialties, obstetrics-gynecology and its subspecialties, and other specialties such as rehabilitation medicine and psychiatry.

Staffing. Teaching hospital clinics are staffed by four categories of physicians. Voluntary attending staff may draw clinic duty as part of their obligation to the hospital for admitting privileges. Full-time, inpatient physicians, usually more junior ones, may be assigned, generally to carry out teaching, supervisory, and research functions. House staffs, usually residents, but occasionally interns, are assigned to clinics on a rotating basis. In most hospitals the stress is on teaching and research rather than on patient care. Since house staffs are usually rotated frequently between various subspecialty clinics for teaching purposes, patients with stable conditions, coming to a subspecialty clinic, say once every three months, may see a different physician each time. Finally, for clinics which are very busy, hospitals may hire outside physicians on a sessional or salaried basis, exclusively to work in the clinics. They are usually not part of the regular hospital staff and do not participate in the educational program. As John Knowles has said of hospital medical staffs: "Those on the 'inside' saw inpatients; the 'outs' worked with the 'outs'" (1965, p. 70).

Patterns of use. Most hospital outpatient departments are open all day every day, but many individual clinics, particularly when they are highly subspecialized, meet once or twice a week. Some teaching hospitals have over a hundred different specialty and subspecialty clinics. Thus, a hospital-based physician working in the usual hospital clinic organization can concentrate on diabetes, peripheral vascular disease, or stroke, in his teaching and/or research. This is advantageous to the physician who has a focus confined to a particular disease or condition. It may also be advantageous to the patient who has a single disease problem which is of a rather complex or unusual nature.

Three kinds of patients face difficulties in using such clinics. One is the patient with the ordinary problem for which no specialty clinic exists. For example, few hospitals have "sore-throat" clinics. Second is the patient with a categorical disease like diabetes, which, however, is uncomplicated. Going to a diabetes clinic, such a patient is likely to have to take a back seat to a diabetic patient who has complications. Third is the patient with multiple problems. These patients, often elderly, may end up attending diabetes clinic on Tuesday, stroke clinic on Wednesday, peripheral vascular clinic on

Thursday, and cardiology clinic on Friday. (Fortunately, Monday is a free day.) This is distinctly disadvantageous for two major reasons: multiple trips to the clinic are necessary and no one can look at the patient as a whole person rather than as a collection of diseased organs and organ systems.

Thus the basic conflict in hospital ambulatory services is established, between the needs of specialty-oriented providers on the one hand and patient with either ordinary problems or several different problems on the other. This situation is not new, and neither is the recognition of it. In 1964, at a conference on "The Expanding Role of Ambulatory Services in Hospitals and Health Departments" held at the New York Academy of Medicine, Cecil Sheps, M.D., said:

> As I sat through the sessions yesterday and today I had a persistent feeling of *déjà vu*. I possess a book [*Clinics, Hospitals and Health Centers*] written by Michael M. Davis and published [by Harper] in 1927. In it there is quoted a statement prepared in 1914 that describes the purpose of an outpatient department just as clearly as anything said at this conference: that the focus must be on the patient, that care must be organized around the patient, and that the hospital must take the community as its venue and not simply the patients who come to it. (Sheps, 1965, p. 148)

At the same conference John Knowles outlined his view of what comprehensive ambulatory care in the hospital setting would mean:

> Comprehensive medicine in this context means the coordination of all the various caring elements in the community with those of the medical profession by a team of individuals representing all disciplines, with all the techniques and resources available to the physician and his patient. The aim of these individuals would be to provide total care—somatic, psychic, and social—to those in need, and to study and research the expanding social and economic problems of medical care with the intent of improving the organization and provision of health services. (Knowles, 1965, p. 73)

As Freymann says, "instead of dividing diagnoses among doctors, doctors should be divided among patients" (1974), p. 255).

The Organization of Hospital Ambulatory Services

There are at least as many modes of organization of hospital ambulatory services as there are types of hospitals. We will examine briefly one of the major patterns of organization that is found in a typical teaching hospital which has both an emergency unit and clinics. In many such hospitals, there are three vertical organizational lines: one for the medical staff, one for the nursing staff, and one for business administration, support services, and hotel operations. (It is interesting to note that *hospital* and *hotel* both derive from the same Latin word.) Sometimes these vertical lines meet in the director's office; sometimes they never meet; occasionally they are well integrated.

This organizational structure is reflected in the ambulatory services. Generally each medical department is responsible for physician services in its own clinics. The pattern may extend to the emergency unit as well, or it may be the primary responsibility of one department, say surgery. Alternatively, physician staffing in the emergency unit may be entirely the responsibility of a separate entity, an Emergency Department, which may stand on its own, may be part of a Department of Ambulatory Services or Community Medicine, or may be attached to the office of the hospital's director. In teaching hospitals, Departments of Ambulatory Services, when they exist, may exert some control over clinic physician staffing.

The Nursing Department generally controls the nursing services for both clinics and emergency units, sometimes designating an associate or assistant director of nursing for ambulatory care. Likewise, the hospital's administration runs the clerical and other support services, often through an associate or assistant administrator or director.

This tripartite approach works well as long as one is not particularly interested in establishing one coordinated *program* in ambulatory care. However, when there is not one person or office in charge of all the resources required to provide ambulatory services, it is very difficult indeed to mount a unified program (Jonas 1973). If one is interested in providing ambulatory services of a comprehensive nature in which the patient, rather than the disease or injury, is the focus, coordination of physician, nursing, and support services under unified leadership is essential.

Possible solutions. Hospitals around the country are wrestling with this problem. Its resolution requires major changes in the way in which hospitals are administratively structured. To do that, some major changes in the way people think and feel will also be required. With a few exceptions, hospitals are not used to mounting co-ordinated *programs,* but rather to delivering *services,* with each component carrying out its functions more or less as its sees fit. To establish an ambulatory care program with a single director having ultimate responsibility for the whole means that the medical, nursing, and support services must each surrender some sovereignty, some-thing each is loathe to do. Furthermore, even if this is done, and a *functionally decentralized* program in ambulatory care offering coordinated, comprehensive care to patients is developed, other problems may be created. Does one end up with duplicated depart-ments of medicine, pediatrics, surgery, nursing, and clerical services for inpatient and outpatient services for the very important func-tions of hiring, firing, discipline, quality control, setting patient-care policies, education, research, and the like? The final answer on this question is not yet in.

Freymann (1974, p. 255) suggested maintaining specialty clinics but requiring them all to become general patient management clin-ics at the same time. Others (Goodrich et al.) have sanctioned the reduction of the number of specialty clinics to the greatest degree possible and creating undifferentiated management clinics in which, for example, internists, regardless of their subspecialty interest, would be required to function as general internists and manage all patient problems.

It is obvious that either approach requires tremendous attitudinal changes on the part of existing hospital medical staffs and adminis-trations which will not be easily forthcoming. In fact, Goodrich et al., with considerable experience in attempting to institute com-prehensive care in several different hospital clinics under several different organizational forms, raised serious questions about wheth-er it could be done at all. That remains to be seen.

It is certain that many of the problems are created by the pres-ent conflicts in the role and work of hospitals between service, teaching, and research as reflected in the contrast between the needs of the majority of patients presenting themselves for care to hospital clinics and the needs of the majority of the physician staffs to carry out their teaching and research functions as they see fit. Presently the latter require a disease orientation, and generally an orientation toward diseases requiring hospitalization at one point or another. If teaching and research were to be reoriented toward an emphasis on the more common rather than on the more uncommon, if hospitals were to define their roles and responsibilities in terms of community needs, as proposed in Freymann's concept of the *mission-oriented hospital* (1974, sec. 5), the conflicts would be resolved straight away, and hospital clinics would be on the road to first-class status (Jonas 1968, 1971).

Medical Education and Problems in Hospital Ambulatory Care

In most United States medical schools, where most physicians who practice in this country receive their training, ambulatory care takes a back seat (Murray, 1972). The bulk of clinical medical education in the United States takes place in short-term general hospitals and concerns the care of inpatients (White, 1973). The bulk of professional training for most other health care professionals takes place in hospitals too. In the course of this training, in most educational institutions students are taught that inpatient care is the most important, the most demanding, the most rewarding, and the most "interesting." Most medical students are heavily exposed to the "interesting case syndrome" by attending physician staffs early in their training. This syndrome appears to be highly contagious. However, most practicing physicians ultimately spend a majority of their time taking care of patients on an ambulatory basis, not in the hospital. In the ambulatory care sector many patients are seen who have health problems which moderately or seriously interfere with their life functioning, but which would never, or hardly ever, require hospitalization: osteoarthritis, low-back pain, mild depression, sexual dysfunction, venereal disease, mild vision and hearing disabilities, skin problems, allergies, and upper respiratory system maladies (National Ambulatory Medical Care Survey, 1975, Tables

3, 4, 7). Furthermore, good ambulatory care, with a large dose of prevention, will very likely reduce the necessity for hospitalization for patients with other conditions potentially requiring hospitalization, like hypertension, diabetes, or a tendency to heart disease (Weinerman, 1965; Comptroller General of the U.S. 1972, p. 762). Nevertheless, despite these facts, it is inpatient care which is stressed in health care professional, particularly physician, training.

There are a variety of reasons to account for the position of ambulatory care in the health care educational system (Freymann, 1974, p. 196). First, the Flexner reforms of the early twentieth century concentrated medical education on the hospital (Freymann, chap. 4). Once control of the medical education system was placed in the hands of hospital-based physicians, they were able to consolidate and then expand their power through their control over resources and their influence over the career choices of each succeeding generation of medical students. The control of the system by hospital-based physicians, and their colleagues, physician and nonphysician, in full-time medical research, was really solidified by the large flow of federal research dollars which went to medical schools in increasing amounts following World War II, reaching its peak in the mid-1960s (Strickland, 1972, p. 248).

Full-time hospital physicians and medical researchers do not have much interest in ambulatory care, primarily because they themselves are the products of the hospital-centered system. Since they control curriculum for both undergraduate and graduate medical education, not much time is spent either on teaching what the physician needs to know to practice good ambulatory care medicine or on teaching in ambulatory care settings. Because of their own training and interests, most medical educators are not very interested in seeing that the various kinds of ambulatory care facilities which are available are attractive places in which to work, teach, or take care of patients.

A second related major factor in determining the relative position of hospital ambulatory care is the private medical practice sector. Private physicians, in their own offices and in hospitals, provide the majority of health care services in the United States. However, because they have been taught in medical school themselves that hospital work is the most important and "interesting" aspect of medical care, many of them downgrade ambulatory care, even their own. Furthermore, once in private practice as individual entrepreneurs, they really don't want to encourage medical school or hospital interference in their practices. Thus in a sense they encourage their own isolation. Further most private practitioners who do hospital work do so in nonteaching hospitals, where there are no full-time physicians except in emergency rooms. They are naturally not eager to see their hospitals establish hospital-based ambulatory services which would be in competition with their practices. Finally, the existence of private practice, with its high-income potential, sharply reduces the pool of physician talent available to work in organized ambulatory care settings as opposed to private practice.

The third major factor in the secondary status of ambulatory care is the United States health care financing system. (Freymann, 1974, chap. 6). It is well known that the current financing system encourages the use of hospital services at the expense of ambulatory care services.

What we have here is a circular process, which is why change is so difficult. In making an analysis, one can start anywhere on the circle. Hospitals provide a great deal of ambulatory care. In terms of patient needs for comprehensive, coordinated, continuous care, they do a relatively poor job. Hospitals, of course, rely on physicians to provide the needed medical services. Most physicians receive most of their training in hospitals, where they are infected with an anti-ambulatory care bias. Hospital medical staffs generally replicate themselves, and full-time private practitioners do little teaching and in any case are generally not interested in "routine" care. Therefore, the new physicians learn from the old ones, and the process goes on apace. One solution is radically new approaches to medical education, a subject with which I deal elsewhere (Jonas, in press).

Hospital Ambulatory Services in New York City

In New York City, it is becoming difficult to distinguish voluntary and municipal hospital outpatient departments by appearance, organization, or function. Most of the large hospitals, whether municipal or voluntary, have teaching functions. Because of population shifts, many of the large teaching voluntaries now find themselves in poor neighborhoods. In the last ten years, the voluntaries have been handling about 50 percent of the hospital outpatient load in the city. Thus, clinics in both groups of hospitals presently carry out similar functions for similar patient populations. Furthermore, voluntary hospitals find themselves deriving their income increasingly from government sources. However, they do run deficits on their outpatient services because significant numbers of patients are not beneficiaries of third-party payment systems. In New York City, in fact, because of the municipal hospital affiliation agreements under which voluntary hospitals and medical schools provide professional staff for the municipal hospitals under contract, the physician staffing patterns of many municipal hospitals look very much like those seen in voluntary hospitals.

The general picture of the contemporary hospital clinic in New York City, whether voluntary or municipal, is as follows. It is heavily populated with patients with common health problems who cannot afford to pay for their own care and who for the most part do not have third-party payment available. The clinics, however, are not generally organized to deal with such patients in a manner most conducive to care which is especially beneficial for them. The historical philosophy is based on charitable obligation and means-testing. Most New York City hospital clinics, whether voluntary or municipal, have many specialty and subspecialty units, usually because of educational and research needs. Although this is useful for the patient who has a sharply defined, single problem, it is not always so useful for the patient whose care may be benefitted most by integration rather than by disintegration. The tendencies of hospital clinics to disintegrate care rather than integrate it are reinforced by their adoption of the traditional tripartite hospital mode of administrative organization.

Into this situation, then, are thrust efforts at quality control, which we will discuss in general in the next chapter. Quality control has not been a major feauture of the United States health care system. Organized ambulatory care has not received a great deal of stress in it either. In the programs which this book considers, two of the stepchildren have been thrown together in different ways. As we will see, the results have been most enlightening.

References

American Hospital Association. *Hospital statistics: 1976 edition.* Chicago, Ill., 1976.

Comptroller General of the United States. *Study of health facilities construction costs.* Washington, D.C.: U.S. Government Printing Office, 1972.

Danchik, K. M. Physician Visits: Volume and interval since last visit— 1971. *Vital and Health Statistics*, Series 10, Number 97. Washington, D.C.: Health Resources Administration. USDHEW, March 1975.

Freymann, J. G. *The American health care system: Its genesis and Trajectory.* New York: Medcom Press, 1974.

Goodrich, C. H., et al. Hospital-based comprehensive care: Is it a failure? *Medical Care*, 1972, *10*, 363.

Jonas, S. *A review of the ambulatory care services of Mount Sinai Hospital, Chicago, Illinois.* Prepared for E. D. Rosenfeld Associates, Inc., New York, N.Y., 1968. Process.

Jonas, S. *Some thoughts on the development of Methodist Hospital of Brooklyn, N.Y.* Prepared for WHK Associates, Inc., New York, N.Y., 1971. Process.

Jonas, S. Some thoughts on primary care: Problems in implementation. *International Journal of Health Services*, 1973, *3*, 177.

Jonas, S., Monitoring utilization of a municipal hospital emergency department. *Hospital Topics*, January/February 1976, p. 43.

Jonas, S. *Medical Education in the United States.* New York: Norton, 1978. In press.

Knowles, J. H. The role of the hospital: The ambulatory clinic. *Bulletin of the New York Academy of Medicine*, 1965, *41*, 2nd Series, 68.

Murray, R. H. The use of technology in ambulatory health care. *Bull. New York Academy of Medicine*, 1972, *48*, 955.

National Ambulatory Medical Care Survey. *Monthly Vital Statistics Report.* Vol. 24, No. 4, Supplement (2), July 14, 1975.

Roemer, M. I. Organized ambulatory health service international perspective. *International Journal of Health Services*, 1971, *1*, 18.

Roemer, M. I. From poor beginnings: The growth of primary care. *Hospitals, J.A.H.A.*, March 1, 1975.

Rosenberg, C. E. Social class and medical care in nineteenth-century America: The rise and fall of the dispensary. *Journal of the History of Medicine and Allied Sciences*, 1974, *29*, 32.

Sheps, C. G. Conference summary and the road ahead. *Bulletin of the New York Academy of Medicine*, 1965, *41*, 2nd Series, 146.

Stevens, R. *American medicine and the public interest.* New Haven: Yale University Press, 1971.

Strickland, S. P. *Politics, science and dread disease.* Cambridge, Mass.: Harvard University Press, 1972.

Weinerman, E. R. Anchor points underlying the planning for tomorrow's health care. *Bulletin of the New York Academy of Medicine*, 1965, 2nd Series, *41*, 1213, 1965.

White, K. L. Life and death and medicine. *Scientific American*, September 1973, *229*: 23.

3

Health Care Quality Measurement and Control

Why Be Concerned with Quality of Care?

A number of measures show that health care delivered in the United States varies sharply in quality. The approaches used to measure and regulate the quality of care aim at ensuring good care. Before beginning to look at some of the efforts which have been undertaken in quality control, we might ask ourselves, "Why be concerned about the quality of health care at all?"

First, perhaps, is the principle *primum non nocere*: "primarily, do no harm." This precept is at least as old as the Hippocratic oath, of which it is a part. This is an important consideration in a health care delivery system in which, as many studies have shown, a substantial minority of care delivered is of less than good quality and could be harmful.

Second, United States society devotes a significant portion of its economic resources to providing health services, and that proportion is increasing. As a result, Americans have a strong interest in obtaining a good product for the money spent. Further, there are social and humanitarian motivations to see that the large sums of money spent actually help those persons who are receiving the services.

About one-half of the material in this chapter is taken from chapter 13, "Quality of Care," which I wrote, in *Health Care Delivery in the United States,* which I edited (New York: Springer Publishing Co., 1977). It is used with the permission of the publisher. Most of the balance of the material comes from the original report, some of which was taken from a paper entitled "PSRO: Issues in Quality Review and Regulation," which I presented at the Annual Meeting of the American Public Health Association, Oct. 22, 1974, in New Orleans, La.

Third, from the providers' point of view, a major motivation for doing good work in health care is professionalism. Like all things, professionalism is a concept which has many internal contradictions. As Freidson demonstrated (1970), arriving at a definition of the term *profession* is a difficult task. The concepts of *profession* and *professionalism* are related to quality. A profession is, in part at least, a field of human endeavor in which the practitioners themselves control entry and exit, in which a common body of knowledge exists, and in which the practitioners attempt to expand and develop that body of knowledge to improve the quality of human life and extend the understanding of man's existence. This last aspect of professionalism, aside from personal pecuniary and self-protective interests, adds a strong impetus to the thrust of at least part of the medical profession to regulate and improve the quality of medical care.

Finally, there is a strong social ethic in our culture to do a good job "for the thing in itself." This seems to be a natural human striving, intangible as that concept may be, to do a good job, of whatever one is doing. Surrounding that basic motivation are cultural influences, which strengthen the striving feelings with ethical and moral imperatives: "Be the best"; "Just being good isn't good enough"; "Winning is everything"; "Everybody loves a winner." Competition is a basic element of American life and culture, indeed of the life and culture of all countries which follow the Judeo-Christian tradition. Being "the best," however that is measured, gets rewarded in business, the professions, the academic world, in athletics. (An interesting observation is that in our society manual labor is one area where being "the best" often doesn't mean too much.)

However, the explanation for the existence of "striving to do a good job" is more basic than that. Striving to do a good job has real survival value and thus, is very explicable in terms of evolutionary theory. The bird which builds a good, safe nest, apparently by instinct, out of which eggs will not fall, is certainly improving the chances of survival of his/her immediate family, and ultimately his/her species, vis-à-vis the bird which builds an unsafe nest. Early men who somehow knew how to find or construct safe habitations, "good" ones that is, were more likely to survive than those who did not. When in modern times one adds the culturally determined ethical, moral, and indeed aesthetic imperatives, which themselves are probably at point of origin related to species survival, to the survival value of "doing a good job," the seemingly intangible "good for the thing in itself" becomes a very strong force indeed. In health care, many measures and procedures have direct individual or species survival value, if they are of good quality. Conversely, the same procedures may have a neutral, or even negative, effect on individual or species survival if done poorly. Examples of this, for the individual, are the removal of an acutely inflamed appendix and, for the species, sanitary water supply. The fact that few if any papers on quality of medical care even bother to discuss the "why" is a strong indication of just how deeply entrenched the feeling is: most writers don't feel the necessity of discuss it, it seems to be so taken for granted.

Can the Quality of Health Care Be Measured?

The extent to which quality of care can be evaluated has been a subject of debate. A former president of the American Medical Association, Russell Roth, said in a presidential address that "good quality in medical care is not something which can be expressed in dollars of cost, hours of time, or, for that matter, in decibels of political oratory. Quality of such medical care is not a tangible qualifiable thing" (*American Medical News*, Dec. 10, 1973). He added there are "immense difficulties" inherent in properly identifying high-quality care.

On the other hand, many authorities in the field have thought it possible to measure and regulate the quality of discrete instances of care delivery. E. A. Codman has been recognized as the originator of outcome studies (C. Lewis, 1974; Christoffel, 1976a; Brook, 1973b, p. 32; Moore, 1975). Emphasizing his faith in their efficacy as measures of quality, Codman said: "While a layman could not authoritatively inquire into the details of the reasons why, he could insist that the end-result system should be used, that someone must see that it is used, and that an efficiency committee be appointed for the purpose" (C. Lewis, p. 800). Lee and Jones wrote a landmark work on quality determination in 1933, which was built around the concept that "good medical care is the kind of medicine practiced and taught by the recognized leaders of the medical profession at a given time or period of social, cultural, and professional development in a community or population group" (1962, p. 6). In 1951, E. R. Weinerman, reflecting the 1949 statement by the Subcommittee on Medical Care of the American Public Health Association, "The Quality of Medical Care in a National Health Program," said: "The quality of medical care is a composite of all the technical, organizational, and financial aspects of any program for personal health service. Good quality can be defined, consciously planned, and evaluated" (Subcommittee on Medical Care, 1949; Weinerman). In their work describing the "tracer method" of quality measurement, David Kessner and his coauthors said (p. 189): "The question is no longer whether there will be intervention in health services to assure quality, but who will intervene and what methods they will use." Finally, in a review article, Robert Brook said: "Even though the perfect system for assessment and assurance of quality of care may not yet exist, innumerable simple efforts can be made to improve quality of care. If applied in a systematic manner, many are likely to be successful" (1973a, p. 133).

Methods of Measuring and Controlling the Quality of Care

To analyze quality control in health care, we must understand the approaches and techniques being used in the United States in this field.[1] The *approaches* are those various methods utilized to ensure quality in the health care delivery system, such as licensing, accreditation, and peer review through hospital medical staff committees. *Techniques* are the ways in which quality is measured within the various approaches. Techniques are only tools; approaches use the tools to effect control, or at least attempt to do so. Thus techniques are scientific constructs whereas approaches are political ones.[2]

1. Many articles (Donabedian, 1966, 1968; Sanazaro and Williamson, 1968; Sheps, 1955; Brook, 1973b, pp. 7–16; Blum, 1974) have established and reviewed the schemata for classifying the techniques used for measuring the quality of medical care delivered by individuals or institutions.
2. In the early 1970s, M. Roemer (1972), Lewis (1974), and Ellwood et al. (1973, chap. 3) began to take this broader view.

APPROACHES TO QUALITY MEASUREMENT AND CONTROL

The approaches may be divided into two groups (Table 3–1): the general and the specific. The general approaches examine and in- dividual's or an institution's ability to meet established evaluative criteria at a particular point in time. Individuals are evaluated in terms of experience, education, and knowledge (usually measured by examination). Institutions are evaluated on the basis of physical structure, administrative and staff organization, minimum services, and personnel qualifications. If the criteria are met at the time of evaluation, it is then predicted that the individual or institution will function well either indefinitely, as in the case of the medical license, or for a given period of time, as in the case of the hospital license. The general approaches used in the United States are licensing, accreditation, and certification (Secretary's Report, 1971).

TABLE 3–1

Approaches, Techniques, and Criteria Used
in the Measurement and Control of the Quality of Care

APPROACHES		TECHNIQUES	CRITERIA
General	*Specific*		
Licensing	Hospital medical staff review committees	Structure	Explicit
Accreditation	Research studies	Process	Implicit
Certification	Professional Standards Review Organization	Outcome evaluation	
	Patient satisfaction		
	Malpractice litigation		

The specific approaches to quality measurement and control, on the other hand, look at discrete instances of provider-patient inter- action—that is, particular examples of the delivery or care—and evaluate them using one of several available techniques. The major specific approaches in use in the United States are hospital medical staff review committees; research studies; Professional Standards Review Organizations; and patient satisfaction, and its subset, mal- practice litigation, an extreme product of patient dissatisfaction.

TECHNIQUES AND CRITERIA FOR QUALITY MEASUREMENT
AND CONTROL

Techniques. Donabedian has provided the generally accepted classification of the techniques of quality assessment (1969, pp. 2–3):

Three major approaches[3] to the evaluation of quality have been identified. These have been designated as the evaluation of structure, process, and outcome or end results. Appraisal of structure involves the evaluation of the settings and instrumentalities available and used for provision of care. While including the physical aspects of facilities and equipment, structural appraisal goes far beyond to encompass the characteristics of the administrative organization and the qualifications of health professionals. . . .

Two major assumptions are made when structure is taken as an indicator of quality: First, that better care is more likely to be provided when better qualified staff, improved physical facilities, and sounder fiscal and administrative organization are employed. Second, that we know enough to identify what is good in terms of staff, physical structure, and formal organization. . . .

Assessment of process is the evaluation of the activities of physicians and other health professionals in the management of patients. The criterion generally used is the degree to which management of patients conforms with the standards, and expectations may be derived from what is considered to be "ideal," "good," or "acceptable" practice as formulated by recognized leaders in the profession. Such standards may also be inferred from patterns of care observed in actual practice. . . .

When evaluation of process is the basis for judgments concerning quality, a major assumption is that health care is useful in maintaining or promoting health. Furthermore, there is the explicit or implicit assumption that particular elements and aspects of care are known to be specifically related to successful or unsuccessful health outcomes or end results. Assessments of outcomes is the evaluation of end results in terms of health and satisfaction. That this evaluation in many ways provides the final evidence of whether care has been good, bad, or indifferent is so

3. Donabedian uses the word *approaches* in the sense in which the word *techniques* is used in this chapter.

because of the broad fundamental social and professional agreement on what results are deemed desirable. Furthermore, it is assumed that good results are brought about, at least to a significant degree, by good care.

Thus, the structural approach examines the setting of care and/ or the qualifications of the providers of care; the process approach examines what goes on between the provider(s) and the patient; the outcome approach examines the results of the encounter or lack thereof between the patient and the health care delivery system. In the main, the structural technique is used in the general approaches, while the process and outcome techniques are used in the specific approaches, sometimes in combination with the structural technique as well.

Criteria. In all three techniques, explicit or implicit criteria are used in the evaluation process. Explicit criteria are written down, and the work under study is checked against them. For example, in a process study of physician performance an explicit criterion might be that in the course of a good physical examination a blood pressure measurement be taken.

Implicit criteria, on the other hand, exist only in the mind of the evaluator. Nothing specific to look for is written down. Evaluators are picked on the basis of their own credentials and reputations. The assumption is made that since they are "good" physicians (or dentists, nurses, etc.), they will know what "good" and "bad" care are and will be able to make valid and reliable assessments of care as they review it.

Thus, there are two groups of approaches, three sets of techniques, and two categories of criteria. They are organized in various combinations in practice in the United States.

Limitations of Widely Used Approaches to Quality Measurement and Control

The structural technique has serious limitations in measuring or estimating the quality of medical care. It has indeed never been shown that there is any relationship between retrospective measurements of the quality of medical care undertaken using structural techniques and those undertaken using process and/or outcome techniques. In fact, the structural technique has fallen into such disfavor as a possible measurement tool that it is not even considered by such contemporary academic investigators of methodological problems in medical care evaluation as Kessner et al. (1973) and Brook (1973), who concerned themselves with the evaluation of process and outcome techniques only.

Just as the structural approach has its limitations in the retrospective evaluation of the quality of medical care, so too does it have its limitations as a predictor of future performance. The basis of evaluation of an individual applicant for a medical license is structural. However, no one has ever shown that there is any relationship between qualifying for a medical license and the quality of the product delivered by the physician or nurse or other licensed health professional over the course of their professional lives, or at any discrete point in time in the future. Indeed, other types of studies of the work of licensed providers, using process and/or outcome techniques, show such a wide variation in quality (Peterson et al.; Morehead et al.: Donabedian 1969; Brook, 1973a, b) that it must be assumed that licensing has very little validity as either a predictor or a guarantor of performance. Nevertheless, of all the available techniques, in the United States it is the structural ones which are the most widely used and the most generally accepted.

This fact applies to institutional licensure, as well. As of 1968, 11 types of medical or residential-care facilities were subject to licensure in the United States (Hollis, pp. 1–20). All or most states required licensing of psychiatric, short- and long-stay hospitals, hospitals and homes for the mentally retarded, nursing and other homes for the aged, and homes for unwed mothers and for dependent children (Hollis, Table A). Structural techniques of evaluation are the rule in institutional as well as individual licensure. The Joint Commission on the Accreditation of Hospitals (JCAH) too limits itself to the use of structural techniques, although one of its new standards does specify that hospitals must engage in process- and/or outcome-oriented medical auditing (Joint Commission, 1976). The JCAH has gone so far as to develop a prototypical medical audit system in great detail. It is called the Performance Evaluation Procedure (PEP) (Fitzgibbon, 1975; Jacobs et al.; Jacobs and Christoffel, 1975).

Donabedian put the case on structural techniques succinctly: "It is generally conceded that the appraisal of structure is too indirect to be definitive" (1969, p. 3).

On the other hand, Christoffel has pointed out that evaluation of structure is not entirely worthless: "While the presence of various input measures in no way assures good care, the converse—good care is unlikely where such inputs are lacking—probably makes sense" (1976b).

As we shall, see, the New York State Health Department confines itself to using the structural approach in dealing with quality of care in hospitals. However, the New York City Health Department has moved into the use of process, as well as the structural, techniques at least in its efforts in quality control under the Ambulatory Care Program. The process method has its limitations, too, as Blum, for example, has pointed out (1974). However, it does look at discrete instances of care delivery and thus represents an advance over using the structural method alone—one of the important findings of this study, as we will see as we examine the efforts in hospital ambulatory care quality control of the New York State and New York City Health Departments.

References

Peers' role stressed by AMA president. *American Medical News,* Dec. 10, 1973, p. 3.

Blum, H. L. Evaluating health care. *Medical Care,* 1974, *12,* 999.

Brook, R. H. Critical issues in the assessment of quality of care and their relationship to HMO's. *Journal of Medical Education, 48,* 114, April 1973, Part 2 (a).

Brook, R. H. *Quality of care assessment: A comparison of five methods of peer review.* National Center for Health Services Research and Development. Washington, D.C.: USDHEW, 1973 (b).

Christoffel, T. Medical Care Evaluation: An Old New Idea. *Journal of Medical Education,* 1976 (a), *51,* 83.

Christoffel, T. Personal communication. March 15, 1976 (b).

Donabedian, A. Evaluating the quality of medical care. *Milbank Memorial Fund Quarterly,* 1966, *44,* 166.

Donabedian, A. Promoting quality through evaluating the process of patient care. *Medical Care,* 1968, *6,* 181.

Donabedian, A. *A guide to medical care administration. II: Medical care appraisal—Quality and utilization.* New York, N.Y.: American Public Health Association, 1969.

Ellwood, P. M., Jr., et al. *Assuring the quality of health care.* Minneapolis, Minn.: Interstudy. 1973.

Fitzgibbon, A. Future of the J.C.A.H. Part II, Joint commission's strengths emerge amid wide criticism. *Hospital Tribune,* May 19, 1975.

Freidson, E. *Profession of medicine.* New York, N.Y.: Dodd, Mead and Company. 1970.

Hollis, G. *State licensing of health facilities.* Rockville, Md.: National Center for Health Statistics, USDHEW, 1968.

Jacobs, C. M., & Christoffel, T. M. *The rationale for outcome audit.* Quality Review Center. Chicago, Ill.: Joint Commission on Accreditation of Hospitals, 1975.

Jacobs, C. M., et al. *Measuring the quality of patient care.* Cambridge, Mass.: Ballinger Publishing Co., 1976.

Joint Commission on Accreditation of Hospitals. *Accreditation manual for hospitals, 1976.* Chicago, Ill.

Kessner, D. M., et al. Assessing Health quality: The case for tracers. *New England Journal of Medicine,* 1973, *288,* 189.

Lee, R. I., & Jones, L. W. *The fundamentals of good medical care.* University of Chicago Press, 1933. Reprinted. Hamden, Conn.: Archon Books, 1962.

Lewis, C. E. The state of the art of quality assessment—1973. *Medical Care,* 1974, *12,* 799.

Moore, F. D. Surgical biology and applied sociology: Cannon and Codman fifty years later. *Harvard Medical Alumni Bulletin,* January–February 1975.

Morehead, M. A., et al. *A study of the quality of hospital care secured by a sample of teamster family members in New York City.* New York, N.Y.: Columbia University School of Public Health and Administrative Medicine, 1964.

Peterson, O. L., et al. An Analytical Study of North Carolina General Practice. *Journal of Medical Education, 31,* December 1956, Part 2.

Roemer, M. I. Controlling and promoting quality in medical care. In Havighurst, C. C., and Weistart, J. C., Eds., *Health care from the library of law and contemporary problems.* Dobbs Ferry, N.Y.: Oceana Publications, 1972.

Sanazaro, P. J., & Williamson, J. W. End results of patient care: A provisional classification based on reports by internists. *Medical Care,* 1968, *6,* 123.

Secretary's report on licensure and related health personnel credentialing. Washington, D.C.: USDHEW, June 1971.

Sheps, M. Approaches to the quality of hospital care. *Public Health Reports,* 1955, *70,* 877.

Subcommittee on Medical Care. The quality of medical care in a national health program. *American Journal of Public Health,* 1949, *39,* 898.

Weinerman, E. R. The quality of medical care. *Annals of the American Academy of Political and Social Science,* Jan. 1, 1951, p. 185.

4

The New York State Health Department and Article 28 of the Public Health Laws of the State of New York

Historical Development of the Law

The Public Health Laws of the State of New York are extensive and complex. They fill over 1,000 pages of text. There are 41 articles dealing with matters ranging from the establishment of a department of health to environmental sanitation and communicable disease control. Articles 28 and 29 establish the powers of the New York Department of Health in relation to hospitals and nursing homes (McKinney's, Articles 28 and 29). Subsequent to the passage of Article 28 in 1965, four related articles were created: 28–A, Nursing Home Companies; 28–B, Hospital Mortgage Loan Construction; 28–C, Nurse Manpower Center; and 28–D, Practice of Nursing Home Administration. Article 29 deals with Hospital Survey, Planning and Review.

The Secretary of State of New York publishes the Official Compilation, Codes, Rules, and Regulations of the State of New York. Volumes 10, A, B, and C cover health matters (Official Compilation). Collectively, this massive document is known as the State Health Code. Within it, chapter 5, containing all the parts in the 700 series, is known as the State Hospital Code. That chapter and parts 600–640 were written to implement Articles 28 and 29.

The present Article 28 is a product primarily of the Folsom Report (Folsom et al.) and is often referred to as the Folsom Act, even though M. B. Folsom was not a member of the legislature. However, Article 28, is not a single law but a collection of many, since it has been amended on a number of occasions (New York State Department of Health, 1971). The term *Folsom Act* should be applied, if used at all, to the principle law establishing Article 28. That law is also known as Chapter 795, Laws of 1965.[1] An act with which Folsom is sometimes confused is the Metcalf-McCloskey Act, Chapter 730, Laws of 1964, which forms the core of the present Article 29, dealing with status and powers of the several Hospital Review and Planning Councils in New York, state and regional, requiring for the first time their approval of new hospital construction.

The Folsom Report (1965) was the product of the Governor's Committee on Hospital Costs, established by Governor Nelson Rockefeller in May 1964 to "(1) study the costs of general hospital care in the State and to make recommendations as to how hospitals may best provide high-quality care at the lowest possible cost and (2) to examine the present apportionment of responsibility among State agencies concerned with hospital care and to make recommendations as to how the responsibility of State government may be most effectively carried out" (Folsom et al., p. 2). After an exhaustive study in which much data was reviewed and many witnesses interviewed, the Committee recommended a nine-point program to moderate, monitor, and meet the cost of hospital care:

(1) Moderating the cost of hospital care by using the hospital and other health facilities more effectively.

(2) Enactment of a State hospital insurance law that would extend coverage to the uninsured, establish minimum standards of protection for hospitalization and related services, and arrange for the financing of such protection.

(3) Revisions in the organization, operation, and regulation of hospital prepayment and insurance plans.

(4) A new system of reporting and monitoring the costs of hospital care.

1. Every law in the State of New York has two reference numbers. One is its article number in the Consolidated Laws. The other is the chapter number which indicates the particular year in which it was passed by the state legislature and signed by the governor. Laws are numbered consecutively as they are passed each year.

(5) Payment by the community as a whole—rather than by patients and by the purchasers of prepayment—of various costs of hospital services to the community.

(6) Full payment of the cost of hospital care rendered to indigent and medically indigent patients.

(7) Grants and loans to replenish and construct more modern and efficient hospitals and other health facilities.

(8) Realignment of responsibilities for hospital care among the agencies of State government.

(9) A breathing period in which the foregoing changes can be put into effect without any, or with only minimal, increases in prepayment rates. (Folsom et al., p. 3)

Detailed proposals were made to implement the nine major recommendations, amounting to over 50 subrecommendations (Folsom et al., pp. 3–11).

Naturally, not all of the recommendations and subrecommendations have been put into law, regulation, and/or policy. In summary, the three principal aims of the legislation which has been developed over the years on the basis of the Folsom Report and subsequent relevant experience (Bernstein, 1975; Cicero, 1975; Fleck, 1975; Garry, 1975; Ingraham, 1966, 1973; Solomon, 1975) are (1) the establishment of a program to regulate the number and type of hospital beds in the State of New York, usually referred to as the "certificate-of-need" program, (actually a further development and strengthening of the program which had been started by Chapter 730, Laws of 1964); (2) the establishment of a State Health Department-controlled program for rate-setting in hospital insurance programs; and (3) the establishment of a State Health Department-controlled, uniform, statewide hospital licensing law, the license to be known as an operating certificate.

Prior to the enactment of Chapter 795, Laws of 1965 (the Folsom Act), control over the establishment of new hospitals and licensing of existing hospitals lay within the State Department of Social Welfare, except that Chapter 730, Laws of 1964, did confer upon the Hospital Review and Planning Councils veto power over the establishment of new hospitals. The basic power had been lodged with the Department of Social Welfare because of the hospitals' history as philanthropic and charitable institutions. One serious problem with this approach was that, as with Medicaid in New York State at present, these powers, which are essentially in the health field, were held not only by a nonhealth agency but were delegated by that agency to the approximately 60 local welfare departments around the state. Article 28 transferred all authority over hospital licensing and establishment from the Department of Social Services to the Health Department, along with an ample staff.

Apparently not everyone in the Department of Social Services was happy with this arrangement. According to David Solomon (1975), then in the Health Department Counsel's Office, on February 1, 1966, the day upon which the new law took effect, the pertinent files from the Department of Social Services were literally and unceremoniously dumped on the steps of the Health Department's offices at 84 Holland Avenue in Albany, from whence Health Department staff lugged them inside. Thus the new program began.

As we noted, the program of Article 28 is threefold: certification-of-need, licensing, and rate-setting. The law is lengthy and complex. Portions of it and other parts of the Public Health Law related to this study are reproduced and/or summarized in appendix 3. Portions of the State Health Code, including relevant portions of State Hospital Code[2] are reproduced and/or summarized in appendix 4. It is important to note that significant powers relating to quality of care are contained in other articles, as well as in Article 28. It is clear from a reading of these various documents that the powers of the Commissioner, the Department, and the Public Health Council,[3] in reference to the measurement and regulation of the quality of medical care, are broad indeed, in the law.

---

2. The Hospital Code is a creation, formally, of the State Hospital Review and Planning Council (Cicero, 1975). The council is an appointed board whose functions are summarized in its title. It is part of the State Health Department. It is technically advisory to the Public Health Council (see fn. 3).

3. The Public Health Council is the equivalent of the Board of Health in New York State. It is the highest health-policymaking body in the state, aside from the Legislature and the Governor. The Commissioner is a member; the others are appointed by the Governor, subject to state senate confirmation. Some of the powers of the Public Health Council and the Hospital Review and Planning Council and the relationships between them will presumably be changed under the Health Planning and Resources Development Act of 1974 (P.L. 93–641).

The Implementation and Effects of Article 28

WHAT WAS SUPPOSED TO HAPPEN

According to the "Declaration of policy and statement of purpose" of Article 28: "Hospital and related services including health-related service of the highest quality, efficiently provided and properly utilized at a reasonable cost, are of vital concern to the public health. In order to provide for the protection and promotion of the health of the inhabitants of the state . . . the department of health shall have the central, comprehensive responsibility for the development and administration of the state's policy with respect to hospital and related services. . . ." What was supposed to happen is thus very clear. The New York State Department of Health was supposed to take over the direction of the state's hospital policy, with the aims of protecting and promoting health for the citizens. To do this, the department was to be concerned with quality, efficiency, "proper utilization," and cost control.

In a paper published on March 15, 1966, six weeks after the State Health Department started to exercise its Article 28 powers, Hollis Ingraham, then Commissioner of Health, summarized the aims of the law as follows:

> Article 28 of the Public Health Law, the statute enacted, gives the Health Department the responsibility to approve the construction of all hospitals, which the Department already does for hospitals constructed with Federal Hill-Burton funds; to require reports on the quality, utilization, and cost of hospital care; and to issue a certificate authorizing the operation of a hospital and the power to inspect hospitals. The Department is also to certify whether rate schedules for hospital services are reasonable related to cost in connection with care paid for by government agencies or hospital service corporations such as Blue Cross. (1966, p. 771)

Ingraham went on to describe how the department was reorganized to carry out its new responsibilities. A Division of Hospital Affairs was created. It had three bureaus: Hospital Certification, Medical Review, and Health Economics. The first was to handle the operating certificate (licensing) functions. Inspections were to be done no less than biennially, through the regional offices. The Bureau of Medical Review was to be "engaged in developing and conducting studies of medical care quality appraisal." The Bureau of Medical Economics, which has become the Division of Health Economics, was to have the rate-setting and rate-regulation responsibilities. The responsibilities for operating the certificate-of-need program were given to the already existing Division of Hospital Review and Planning, which at that time had charge of the state's Hill-Burton program. At the same time, the department was also taking up new functions in utilization review and quality control thrust upon it by the advent of Medicare and Medicaid.

This constitutes what is known, publicly at least, about the aims of Article 28. However, although the department was given these broad responsibilities in institutional licensing, rate-setting, and facilities planning, no specific goals were set. Nor were any baselines defined. Thus, no method for evaluating the program itself was built into it. No one said, "These are the numbers and types of hospitals and beds which we have now, and these are the numbers which we would like to have in five years, for the following reasons." No one said, "These are the specific deficiencies in the state's short- and long-term care institutions with which the operating certificate program is intended to deal, over the next five years." The same applies to the rate-setting function. Broad goals in terms of "quality" and "efficiency" were set out, but neither specific objectives, nor even methods of developing specific objectives, were defined, and never have been. Numerators were discussed, but denominators never were. This situation makes evaluating the effects of Article 28 difficult.

WHAT HAS HAPPENED IN GENERAL

No comprehensive reviews or evaluations of Article 28 activities, carried out either by the department itself or outside observers, are available. The Annual Reports of the State Department of Health are not particularly revealing. They are rather skimpy documents, averaging 15 pages for the years 1969 and 1971–1973 (NYS Dept. of Health 1970, 1972, 1973, 1974). The 1969 Annual Report (1970, pp. 2–4) reported the number of construction plans reviewed, the number of beds in health-related facilities certified, the numbers of institutions surveyed for operating certificates and for Medicare approval, the number of existing nursing homes closed and new ones certified, and so on. It also mentioned increased rate-setting and cost-control powers given to the department. In the 1971 Annual Report (1972, p. 3) there is brief mention of Article 28 activities, concerning nursing home audits and health facilities financing. This brevity was matched in the 1972 Annual Report (1973, pp. 9, 17) with a few sentences about the number of new construction and renovation applications received, health-facilities financing activities, and nursing home inspections with particular regard to fire safety. A similar picture is seen in the 1973 Annual Report (1974, p. 10). It is hard to tell from the Annual Reports what the department is actually doing in this area, and it is impossible to make any estimation of the meaning of that activity.

In 1973, Ingraham put out a small pamphlet entitled *The Article 28 Story: Landmark in Health Facility Planning*. Most of its eight pages are concerned with describing the program. Its brief "Results" section is here quoted in full.

New York State's program of mandatory health facility planning went into effect in February 1966.

Based on the results of the first six years of the program, it is estimated that a projected statewide need for 87,000 general care beds and 117,000 long-term care beds of high quality will be fully met by 1977.

During the first six years, the State Health Department received and processed over 3,400 applications seeking permission to establish 136,000 beds and 600 ambulatory care projects.

Of that total, the Department approved proposals to add over 83,000 beds. For various reasons, primarily a considered lack of need, the Department disapproved construction of 51,000 beds— thus saving approximately $1.6 billion in capital costs and $738 million annually in unnecessary operating cost.

Since the law took effect, 38 non-conforming hospitals and 281 non-conforming nursing homes have been closed. Nearly 2,000 maternity beds in hospitals throughout the State have been closed or converted to other, more needed, uses.

In the two years in which the Health Department has had authority to monitor costs and charges, the rate of increase in hospital and nursing home costs has been significantly slowed. Within one year the increase in Medicaid rates declined from 19.1 percent (in 1970) to 10.2 percent (in 1971). In some areas of the State this rate dropped to 5 percent in 1972.

In general, a comparison of New York's present health care picture with that of the nation as a whole, where development has been largely uncontrolled over the same period, shows that the State's mandatory health facility planning program has resulted in:

—construction of fewer, larger, and more efficient health facilities, with a simultaneous reduction in the number of small inefficient inpatient facilities

—improved use rates by the population and more efficient levels of occupancy

—creation of alternate levels of care for lower operating costs and more appropriate placement of patients

—improved availability, quality of care and structural conformity in all facilities throughout the State. (p. 8)

This piece contains the first mention of goals, "87,000 general care beds and 117,000 long-term care beds of high quality . . . by 1977," and of a denominator, "the nation as a whole." However, the basis for the numbers of beds, the definition of "high quality," and the measures used to determine what is going on in "the nation as a whole" are not revealed. If there were any detailed studies giving the rationales for these claims, they were not given to us. The claim on the effectiveness of the cost-control program ignores the coincident existence of the federal Economic Stabilization Program.

Following his election as Governor of New York in November 1974, Hugh Carey established a number of task forces to review the operations of the state government. The Task Force on Health issued a report in December 1974 which draws heavily on the Ingraham pamphlet, both for its description of the program and for the conclusions which it draws.

Thus, it may be concluded that, based on information made available to us or which we could find in the literature or elsewhere, no one really knows, even in general terms, what the impact of Article 28 has been, either on the quality of medical care specifically, or on the aspects of the health care delivery system with which it deals. It should be noted that, according to Fleck (1975), the department has always interpreted its powers in relation to the quality of medical care very narrowly. "Narrow" would sometimes seem to mean "virtual inaction." As long ago as 1963, in Article 2, the Commissioner was empowered to "cause to be made such scientific studies in research which have for their purpose . . . the improvement of the quality of medical audits within the state" (Chap. 326, L. 1963). There is little evidence that anything has been done with this power. As far as the Section 2803 powers are concerned (appendix 3), Fleck said that the department has interpreted "the power to inquire into the operation of hospitals and to conduct periodic inspections of facilities with respect to . . . standards of medical care . . ." (Sec. 2803 [1]) to be limited to a Joint Commission of the Accreditation of Hospitals type of inspection of hospital medical staff organization. As to the powers given to the Public Health Council under Sec. 2803 (2) to "adopt and amend rules and regulations, *subject to the approval of the commissioner* [my emphasis], to effectuate the provisions and purposes of this article, including but not limited to (a) the establishment of requirements for a uniform statewide system of reports and audits relating to the quality of medical and physical care provided . . . ," Fleck said that the Council has never carried out this responsibility, and, in effect, that this was "their problem."

There was, of course, a Bureau of Medical Review established under Article 28 for the purpose of carrying out the quality of care review responsibilities, as noted by Ingraham. It did carry out some discrete studies but never developed any general systems for medical care evaluation. Nor did it establish any systems for evaluating the operations under Article 28 itself. It was abolished in a budget cut in the early 1970s.

The general picture of what was done under Article 28 is thus rather murky, expect that very little has been done with the medical care quality control powers. We will now turn to a consideration of what has happened with the major powers individually.

WHAT HAS HAPPENED WITH CERTIFICATION-OF-NEED

The literature concerning certification-of-need programs is not extensive. It has been reviewed by O'Donoghue et al. (1974, chap. 4, pp. 175–80) and Rothenberg (1975). The major point made by Rothenberg is that little of the literature actually deals with evaluation of certification-of-need experiences. Dorsey published a useful summary of the basic concepts of certification of need (1973). He says that he strongly supports the idea, but does his use of an abbreviation (CON) in referring to certificate-of-need programs, perhaps reveal unconscious thoughts? Cohen raises for consideration certain theoretical problems inherent in the certificate-of-need at great length (1973). Havighurst generally opposes the approach, but his piece is required reading for anyone seriously interested in the subject, if only for its comprehensive review of the medical and legal literature in the whole area of health facilities planning and of the problems of governmental regulation in general. Havighurst has also published a brief summary of his *Virginia Law Review* piece (1974a). He summarized his reservations concerning certification-of-need:

> The circumstances giving rise to my doubts are as follows: (1) The political influence of the hospital industry in the health planning and certification-of-need process; (2) the lack of political pressure to do more than slow down the rate of cost increases—which means that political processes can at best merely stabilize the percentage of GNP devoted to health care, even though a substantial fraction of those billions might be better spent by society on other things; (3) the general implicit belief in the value of more and better health services of all kinds so long as obvious duplication is avoided, a belief which is shared not only by providers and health planners but also by so-called consumers who may be involved in the regulatory process but who will have no occasion to count directly the costs of new or improved services; (4) the actual and potential opportunities for using "internal subsidies"—funds generated by charging monopoly prices for certain popular services—to provide other services which would not be purchased if priced at cost; (5) the orientation of health planners and regulators, not to planning of a technocratic variety, but to incremental change based on consensual processes and political bargaining; and (6) the difficulty of reconciling the need for a substantial contraction in the hospital industry with regulators' naturally protective attitude toward the regulated firms' investments and revenues.

Havighurst, however, is dealing with theoretical constructs, not practical experience. Havighurst edited a report of a conference on the regulation of health facilities construction held in 1972 which contains a number of useful historical, theoretical, and descriptive papers (1974b). Curran's paper (Havighurst 1974b, pp. 85–111) describes certification-of-need laws as they existed in 20 states in 1972.

A few field evaluations of certification-of-need programs have been attempted. In 1972, the General Accounting Office published a massive study of construction costs for health facilities (Comptroller General of the U.S., 1972). In 1974, after review of then available information, O'Donoghue et al. concluded that "there is no evidence supporting the effectiveness or efficiency of capital expenditures regulation. On the other hand, it is equally true that there is no evidence indicating that such regulation is ineffective or inefficient" (1974, p. 4). Bicknell and Walsh examined the first 19 months of experience with certification-of-need in Massachusetts (1975). They described the processes, drew some lessons from the experience, and concluded that it is "no panacea; alone, it is not equal to its broad assignments." Rothenberg (1975, p. 48) referred to an unpublished work by Leavy dealing with the first five years of experience with certification-of-need under Article 28 (1972). Leavy concluded, as quoted by Rothenberg (1975, p. 164), that:

> the improvements and changes in the quantity and quality of the supply of health facilities . . . over the first five years of the operation of Article 28 is due in large measure to selective approval of the construction of 15,499 totally conforming hospital beds, 35,957 long-term care or nursing home beds. . . .

However, Rothenberg points out, Leavy had no control group or period. Several major trends which were noted by him as occurring under Article 28 during 1965–70, such as the reduction in the number of small hospitals, had actually begun by 1960 and were more pronounced during 1960–65 than they were during 1965–70 (1975, pp. 165–166). Leavy, in fact, appears to have been suffering from the "no-denominator" problem which is experienced by the New York State Health Department, as already pointed out.

Rothenberg herself has made what appears to be the first attempt to objectively evaluate certification-of-need under Article 28 to try to determine what it has meant to the development of health services in New York State. She compared the experience on several parameters for the five years preceding the enactment of Ar-

ticle 28 with the experience in the five years following the enactment of Article 28, using various statistical techniques. Two major
questions were asked:

1. What has been the impact of certification-of-need on the rate
   and pattern of change in the number of hospital and health
   care facilities available to the population in selected areas of
   the state?
2. Has the certification-of-need program helped planning agencies
   achieve end results which are closer to desired outcomes than
   was the case before its implementation? (1975, p. 160)

Rothenberg concluded that on the parameters measured, such
as the reduction in the number of hospitals, the increase in hospital
size, and the reduction in the number of small, short-term general
hospital as a proportion of all hospitals, "little could be attributed
to the introduction in 1965 of the certificate-of-need legislation to
regulating hospital bed expansion" (1975, p. 162). Rothenberg comes
to this conclusion because the trends observed under Article 28
were actually well underway before the enactment of the legislation. She also found that "hospitals were more responsive to community need for general care beds before the law than afterwards"
(1975, p. 169). On the other hand, she states, "fewer general care
beds had been added in the twenty-five study counties during the
five years after implementation than during the five years before.
This is especially important because of the potential for a building
boom in short-term general hospitals following enactment of the
Medicare legislation in 1965. . . . Moreover, after 1965, increases in
general care beds tended to occur mainly in counties identified at
the beginning of that time interval (1965–1970) as having a number
of non-conforming beds" (1975, p. 177). However, "general care
beds appeared to be added in areas where either population change
was negative or where it was relatively stable" (1975, p. 178).

Thus, one must conclude from the first quantitative analysis of
the experience with certification-of-need under Article 28 that the
results are a mixed bag at best and may be, at worst, negative. It
is interesting that Andrew Fleck, who was closely associated with
the original development of Article 28 and who has been very much
concerned with the whole question of health facilities capital forma-
tion since that time, stated flatly that certification-of-need "doesn't

work" (1975). He attributes this, not to any fault in the concept, but to serious problems which the State Health Department has had resulting from pressure exerted by parties interested in hospital expansion: hospitals, bankers, builders, philanthropists, and their political representatives. Although the figures are not too meaningful in the absence of information on population changes and geographical distribution, it is interesting to look at what has happened to the raw numbers of short-term beds in New York State in the period 1965–74 (Table 4–1). The overall total has dropped by about 3,500, but there has been an increase of over 4,000 medical-surgical beds.

While there is now some evidence that certification-of-need in New York State has not even worked well as a program, still, no one has even begun to look quantitatively at the question of whether or not certification-of-need is related either to health care costs or to the quality of medical care.[4]

WHAT HAS HAPPENED WITH RATE-SETTING

There are no studies available on the efficacy of rate-setting under Article 28 in relation either to hospital costs or to the quality of medical care. Ingraham made certain claims for New York State's rate-setting efforts (1973). As pointed out, however, there were no controls to account for the possible relationship between the decrease in the rate of increase of hospital costs in New York State in the early 1970s and the presence of the Economic Stabilization Program. However, a study done for the United States Department of Health, Education, and Welfare concluded that rate regulation is useful (Morris Associates, 1975). The conclusion is based on a survey of rate regulation in 24 states. The report said: "The effectiveness of rate review programs is not yet conclusively demonstrated but there is sufficient evidence to suggest the federal government should promote the adoption of even non-binding rate review in every state."

4. In a comprehensive study published in 1977, David Salkever and Thomas Bice found that "[certificate-of-need] legislation has diverted rather than checked hospital capital investments and has therefore had negligible impact on patient costs" ("Impact of State Certificate-of-Need Laws on Health Care Costs and Utilization," Rockville, Maryland: *NCHSR Research Digest Series*, HRA 77-3163, 1977).

TABLE 4-1

Changes in New York State Acute Care Beds, 1965–74

Type of bed	1965 Supply	Closed	Opened	Converted to:						1974 Supply
				Med.-Surg.	Ped.	OB	TB	ICU-CCU[a]	Other	
Medical-surgical	60,609	3,594	8,039	—	—	12	—	29	37	64,976
Pediatric	7,806	773	407	158	—	—	—	9	13	7,260
Obstetrical	8,517	2,626	349	275	4	—	—	—	2	5,959
Other	10,994	4,892	129	32	—	—	—	6	—	6,193
Total	87,926	11,885	8,924	465	4	12	—	44	52	84,388

SOURCE: Fleck, A. C. "Health Care Cost Containment." Presented at Western Regional Health Forum, San Francisco, Calif., Dec. 1–4, 1974. Process.
[a]Intensive Care Unit/Coronary Care Unit.

WHAT HAS HAPPENED WITH THE OPERATING CERTIFICATE PROGRAM

This program provides the major mode of potential impact on the quality of medical care by the State Health Department, aside from the general powers which the Commissioner and the Public Health Council have under Article 28. Once again, there have been no overall evaluations of either the implementation of the operating certificate program or of the relationship between it and the quality of medical care. As indicated by the State Health Department Annual Reports and the Ingraham article (1973), the Health Department tends to review its operating certificate activities simply in terms of visits made and beds approved or closed, whether for hospitals or for nursing homes.

Since the fall of 1974, the nursing home industry in New York State has received a great deal of publicity in the press, as has the relationship of the State Health Department to the industry. Since 1970 the bulk of State Health Department inspectorial activity under the operating certificate program has been concerned with nursing homes, with hospitals not receiving too much attention (Cicero, 1975). However, all that the department can point to in terms of the effects of the program is the closings of homes. For example, in 1975, prior to June 3, "22 unsafe nursing homes had [been] closed . . . , 15 were closing and 44 were awaiting hearings or court appeals" (37 Nursing Homes, 1975). From what has been discovered by numerous investigations of nursing homes, not only presently but in the past as well, it is likely that these closings are entirely necessary, to eliminate pestholes. However, what relationship, if any, such closings have to the overall quality of care received by the population of persons occupying such homes in the state or any of its regions is unknown. The question is not even being asked, but if licensing of institutions is really going to be evaluated, the question must be asked. The other major question is what effect, if any, licensing has on those institutions the majority of which retain their licenses? For the majority of hospitals, does licensing make any difference in the quality of their product, or would they do just as well, or poorly, without it?

Because of the nursing home situation and the limitations on the size of its staff during the 1970-75 period, the Department was not able to come anywhere near meeting the two-year cycle for hospital inspections in New York City mandated by law. In 1975, David Pomrinse, Director of the Mount Sinai Hospital, was unable to recall the last Article 28 inspection of that hospital. "We just send in the papers," he said, "and the operating certificate is automatically renewed." Since 1973, the State Health Department had taken to accepting JCAH reports in lieu of all or part of the inspection necessary for operating certificate renewal (Cicero, 1975; NYS Dept. of Health, Aug. 3, 1973).

In light of this situation, the Consumer Commission on the Accreditation of Health Services has said:

> The New York State Health Department (NYSHD) is required by Public Health Law to inspect hospitals. For the past two years, NYSHD has not fully complied with Article 28 which requires complete hospital inspections every two years before an operating certificate is issued to a hospital. The failure of the NYSHD to meet its mandated legislative responsibility places in jeopardy the life and safety of hospital patients in this state. (Consumer Comission, 1974b, p. 1)

However, how do we really know that lack of inspection "places in jeopardy the life and safety of hospital patients in this state"? It may well do so, but one cannot be at all sure. Another Consumer Commission publication presented two hospital reports which revealed very bad conditions (Consumer Commission, 1974a). They exist in spite of the inspection program, however, and, in the absence of any evaluation of the relationship of the operating certificate program to quality of care, the commission's statement quoted above is unjustified.

Finally, regardless of the degree of efficacy of the operating certificate programs, whatever the standards of measurement adopted and whatever the frequency of inspections, the department is operating with one big disadvantage (Bernstein, 1975). Its *only* real weapon is decertification. When one tries to swat a fly on a table with a sledgehammer, one of three things often happens: one misses, one breaks the table, one declines to swing. Rarely does one kill the fly. Thus the sledgehammer, although a mighty weapon, becomes completely ineffective. In relation to the many flies which one finds as hospital deficiencies, as of 1975 the department found itself equipped only with a sledgehammer.

WHAT HAS HAPPENED TO AMBULATORY CARE QUALITY CONTROL

The provisions of Article 28 concerning quality control in ambulatory services are implemented through the Hospital Code part of the Health Code. The relevant portions of the Hospital Code, Part 703 and Sections 720.17 and 720.18, are summarized in appendix 4. It should be pointed out that the ambulatory care provisions of the code apply only to care given in organized settings, not in private doctors' offices. Because of the large number of hospital clinics in New York City, it is probable that in New York State a higher proportion of total ambulatory care is given in organized settings than in most other states.

Nevertheless, it may be assumed that the proportion of total visits provided in private doctors' offices still approaches the national average of 80 percent (Tenney et al., 1974, p. 2), particularly because of the high doctor/patient ratio experienced by this state. Thus, even if the ambulatory care provisions of the code were to be fully applied, the bulk of ambulatory care in the state would remain unregulated. With all of these limitations, however, we are still interested in Article 28 implementation in reference to ambulatory care.

Despite the fact that we were able to gather direct evidence concerning the experience of certain voluntary hospitals in New York City only, there are several reasons why we believe that the evidence which we gathered in those hospitals is representative of what has happened in the state as a whole. In New York State, aside from emergency services, there are only a few hospitals outside of New York City which provide a significant volume of ambulatory care. In comparison with the volume of service provided by hospital ambulatory services in the state, the volume provided in other organized ambulatory settings is small. The voluntary hospitals which we visited are fairly representative of the voluntary group in the city. There is no reason to believe that the experience in relation to Article 28 enforcement in the New York City municipal hospitals differs from that of the voluntaries. Finally, and most importantly, the picture which we derived of activity vis-à-vis ambulatory care under the provisions of Article 28 based upon our interviews at the selected hospitals did not differ from the picture which was given to us by the official of the New York State Department of Health who has the responsibility for implementing the Hospital Code. Thus, we feel that our understanding represents reality. Activity under Article 28 in relation to ambulatory care is virtually non-existent.

Benjamin Wainfeld, M.D., has been Director of Community Medicine at the Brookdale Hospital since 1971. For the seven years prior to that, he was in ambulatory care at the Maimonides and Coney Island Hospitals in Brooklyn, N.Y. He is past president of the Association of Directors of Ambulatory Care of New York City and is the current president of the Public Health Association of New York. He was involved in the drafting of Sections 720.17 and 720.18 of the Hospital Code. To his knowledge, these sections have never been applied in an operating certificate inspection in a New York City hospital. He has never been personally involved in such an inspection, nor has he ever heard one discussed in settings in which JCAH and ACP inspections are routinely discussed (1975). This view was confirmed by Stanley Reichman, M.D., (1975) of the Hospital for Joint Diseases, Alden Hammerling (1975) of the Roosevelt Hospital, and several other Directors of Ambulatory Care who did not care to be quoted. Gilbert Bernstein (1975) and David Pomrinse, M.D., (1975), both of whom have had extensive experience with hospital affairs in the city of New York, agreed with this view of the situation.

Frank Cicero, M.D., Deputy Commissioner and Director of the Division of Hospital Affairs of the State Department of Health also agreed with this view (1975), as did Jane Garry (1975) who is Director of the Department's Bureau of Ambulatory Care. In the context of the overall responsibilities of the Department under Article 28, and because of the emphasis which nursing home inspections have received in the last five years, implementation of the ambulatory care provisions of the Code have not been given any attention. Cicero did not feel that this is due to a shortage of staff, but rather to a lack of focus. In 1973, the State Health Department decided that ambulatory care should indeed receive some attention, and thus a Bureau of Ambulatory Care was established. The objective of the Bureau is to coordinate and focus the Department's activities in relation to all loci of organized ambulatory care. One major responsibility is to provide guidance in implementation of the ambulatory care provisions of the Hospital Code to the Regional Offices whose responsibility it is to actually carry out the inspections.

Cicero pointed out that ambulatory care was not mentioned at all in the Folsom Act. In the early years of Article 28 development, the department concentrated on getting the total program under way and implementing its major responsibilities in the certificate-of-need and rate-setting programs. In the period 1970–75, in terms of operating certificate inspections, the department had to concentrate heavily on nursing homes. As of the spring of 1975, the bureau hoped to begin field activities in ambulatory care "soon." Thus, the historical picture of the enforcement of ambulatory care standards under Article 28 shows that nothing has happened.

The Causes of Inaction

LIMITED USE OF BROAD POWERS

To review briefly, we were able to find no evidence that the broad powers concerning the quality of medical care granted to the State Commissioner of Health and the Public Health Council under Article 2, Sections 206 and 225, and Article 28, Section 2803, of the Public Health Laws have ever been used to more than a very minor degree. The obligation of the Commissioner to "cause to be made such scientific studies and research which have for their purpose the reduction of morbidity and mortality and the improvement of the quality of medical care through the conduction of medical audits within the state" was carried out for a time, to a limited extent, by the Bureau of Medical Review, but it was closed down in the early seventies as an economy measure. We are not sure what the bureau did, but one measure of its success and influence or lack thereof is that the State Department of Health did not have any summary written material on its work to produce for our consideration.

The question that of course arises is why have the broad Article 2 and 28 powers not been implemented? In answering this question, we have limited hard information to go on. We do have surmises and opinions, however. First of all, it appears as if there has been a general lack of will in the State Health Department to use its legislated authority. Part of this has to do with interpretation of the statute. For instance, we pointed out that Fleck interprets Section 2803 (1) narrowly and, as for Section 2803 (2), he said that that was the Public Health Council's responsibility.

Part of it may have to do with the historical reluctance of Health Departments to tangle with organized medicine. The struggle which Commissioner of Health Herman Biggs had in the 1920s with the State and County Medical Societies over departmental involvement in treatment medicine (described in the next chapter) was not an isolated event. During the period, health departments all over the country fought, and lost, struggles with the organized representatives of private practice to implement C.-E. A. Winslow's definition of *public health*:

> Public health is the science and the art of preventing disease, prolonging life, and promoting physical health and efficiency through organized community efforts for the sanitation of the environment, the control of community infections, the education of the individual in principles of personal hygiene, the organization of medical and nursing service for the early diagnosis and preventive treatment of disease, and the development of the social machinery which will ensure to every individual in the community a standard of living adequate for the maintenance of health. (Winslow, 1920)

Instead, they were left with Haven Emerson's "Basic Six," the functions which he deemed to be appropriate for public health departments: public health laboratories, vital statistics, communicable disease control, environmental sanitation, maternal and child health, and public health education. Since then, health departments have been sensitized. Most people do not like being beaten over the head, and health departments are not unlike most people in this respect. In this regard, notice the care and circumspection with which the Ghetto Medicine legislation was introduced and passed, as described in the next chapter. Nonimplementation of the general quality powers in the Public Health Laws of the State of New York certainly avoided any potential struggle over that issue.

Further in the analysis of why the broad quality powers have not been used, it appears as if the Health Department simply had too much to do with a limited staff. This is apparent, as we will discuss further, with the specific Article 28 powers. The Public Health Laws are voluminous, as are the accompanying codes and the various manuals (internal departmental administrative guides). It is impossible to do everything, unless a conscious political decision is made at the highest political levels (above the Health Department) at which such decisions are made, to put on enough staff and back them up. Thus, with limited staff, choices have to be made.

Finally, the Health Department may well have been law-suit conscious and subject to political pressure. As has become well known during the 1974–76 nursing home scandal investigations, the department had been concentrating its efforts in quality control on the nursing home industry since about 1970. For its efforts, it has been sued innumerable times. The practical results of this are noteworthy. The industry can sue as often as it wishes, on the most frivolous of issues. It has the proverbial battery of lawyers to prosecute its suits, until recently paid for by Medicaid money. The department, in defending itself, must depend on its own hard-pressed Counsel's office and the State Attorney General's office, both thinly staffed in relation to the work load. It may well be that the department figured, either consciously or unconsciously, that it had enough litigation on its hands and did not want to chance inviting more by beginning to implement its broad quality-control powers. Also, the nursing home situation subjected the department to intense political pressure from elected and nonelected officials of both major political parties. The department may well have been attempting to avoid more of the same in choosing not to get into major campaigns on the quality issue. There are very powerful professional, institutional, and religious organizations which might not be anxious to see the department playing a large role in quality control.

SPECIFIC LIMITATIONS OF ACTION

One of the most impressive results of our exploration into the implementation of Article 28 has been the discovery of the virtual lack of literature dealing with the whole subject area. Here we have a major effort by one of the most complex state governments in the country into hospital licensing, certification-of-need, and rate-setting, which has been going on for nearly ten years, and few people have looked at it, at least for publication. This is fascinating, especially since so much public policy nationally, particularly in relation to certification-of-need, has been made on the basis of the New York State legislation. Evaluation needs to take place on two levels. First, how have the programs been implemented? Is what is called for in the law and the regulations actually being done? Enforcement, particularly of the operating certificate program, appears to be very spotty. Is this really true and, if so, why? Second, are the various programs doing what they set out to do? Are they doing anything at all? The Rothenberg study (1975) was the first attempt to study certification of need quantitatively, with any kind of controls. No one has ever looked at the operating certificate program to see, first, if it makes any difference in the levels to which hospitals meet the required structural standards (how many hospitals would meet reasonable standards, anyway?) and, second, if meeting those standards makes any difference insofar as the quality of medical care is concerned. No one has ever looked at the rate-setting program in a controlled manner to see if it makes a difference in rate changes in the state.

Although we admittedly did not interview a broad cross section of the Health Department leadership, among those we did interview, with one exception, we found a rather disturbing lack of knowledge of the academic approach to the general question of program evaluation and to the particular question of measuring the quality of medical care. People were not familiar with the terminology, much less the literaure. At the same time, it should be noted that most of the quality of care literature shows an appalling lack of understanding on the part of the academic community of the problems of the people who have day-to-day responsibility for the implementation of practical quality control programs. Most academic papers in the field offer little help. The real world/academic chasm is deep and wide. This is unfortunate because there are good, smart, well-intentioned people on both sides who, if they could work together, could offer the public a great deal.

Nevertheless, the apparently limited knowledge of evaluative techniques and their importance on the part of State Health Department leadership may well be the reason that the department has done little evaluation of Article 28 itself, except to say, on occasion, that Article 28 is great because so many beds were certified or decertified, so much construction was prevented, so many nursing homes were closed. However, as pointed out above, in terms of the health and health care needs of the people of the state, no program goals were ever defined for the Article 28 program. Further, there are no denominators. We don't know how many of the total number of nursing homes were closed, and we don't know what the closings mean in relationship to the needs of the people of New York State for long-term care. Thus, there is no real basis for the design of the program beyond the feeling that "something has to be done" about bad nursing homes or hospital overbuilding or rapidly rising health care costs.

These findings have obvious national implications. Are we going to have more legislation drawn up on the basis of hunches, surmises, and political needs of certain legislators and executives? Once the legislation is passed into law, is it going to remain unevaluated, or is it going to have meaningful evaluation built into it? It should be obvious by now that meaningful evaluation is not just a pleasant academic exercise, but can have real effects on both cost and quality/cost-benefit. Further, we discussed the limitations of structural standards in chapter 3. The operating certificate program is based on the structural technique of quality evaluation. Thus, even if it were completely implemented, which our evidence has shown it is not, it would be of questionable value.

The discussion of the relationship between Article 28 and the quality of medical care in hospital outpatient departments, one of the two major foci of this study, is, of necessity, brief. The evidence shows that the articles of the Hospital Code relating to hospital ambulatory simply have not been implemented. The State Health Department, until very recently, has not seen ambulatory care as a priority. Frank Cicero, who has responsibility for the operating certificate program among other things, refused, despite repeated prodding, to say that the department needs more staff. But he did say that for several years most of his inspectors have been tied up with the nursing home situation.

Facts are not available on the situation regarding the staffing for facilities inspection, but at a budget hearing in 1970 (Senate Finance Committee, 1970), Deputy Commissioner Klepak stated that the State Controller said that the department could not carry out its fiscal audit responsibilities because of inadequate staff. The next year at a budget hearing (Senate Finance Committee 1971), it was noted that 228 of 1,100 central office positions were vacant. In 1974 (Senate Finance Committee 1974), it was pointed out that the department had available two financial auditors to examine all of the hospitals in the state.

Thus, a combination of an admitted lack of interest and a probable staff shortage has led to the State Health Department's lack of enforcement of hospital ambulatory care standards under Article 28.

THE ROLE OF THE STATE LEGISLATURE

Finally, in discussing the limitations of the Articles 28 program, one must consider the role of the state legislature. This is the body which created, in theory at least, Article 28 and, indeed, the Department of Health. It is the body which, collectively, is supposed to be closest to "the people" and which is supposed to represent "the people's" interest.

There is no record of legislative hearings ever being conducted concerning the performance of the Department of Health in implementing specific Article 28 programs or in carrying out its general quality control responsibilities under Articles 2 and 28. Between 1966 and 1970 there existed a body called the Joint Legislative Committee on the Problems of Public Health, Medicare, Medicaid, and Compulsory Health and Hospital Insurance, chaired by State Senator Norman Lent. None of its four Annual Reports mentioned Article 28 (Joint Legislative Committee 1967, 1968, 1969, 1970). Herbert Miller was the Chairman of the State Assembly Health Committee during the 1975–76 New York State legislative session. By that time, he had been a member of the assembly for about ten years. My interview with him concerning legislative oversight of the operations of the State Health Department went roughly as follows (Miller, 1975):

JONAS Have you ever held hearings on Article 28 or the "Ghetto Medicine" program?

MILLER No.

JONAS What do you think about the performance of the State Health Department in carrying out its responsibilities under Article 28?

MILLER No comment. Look, there is a new Commissioner. I don't want to say anything about him.

JONAS Okay, what do you think about the past performance of the Department in carrying out its Article 28 responsibilities?

MILLER No comment.

JONAS What do you think about the Ghetto Medicine program?

MILLER No comment.

JONAS Do you think that the legislature has a role to play in overseeing the activities of state agencies?

MILLER Our major responsibility is considering proposals for new legislation. If you would like to make some proposals for new legislation, please put them in writing and we will be very happy to consider them. I will not be drawn into a discussion of the actvities of State agencies.
[End of interview]

A tape recorder was not used in the interview, and the above is not direct quotation but paraphrase. Nevertheless, the gist is correct. The public interest in overseeing the activities of the State Health Department is not being protected by the legislature.[5]

Summary

In considering the activities of the State Department of Health under Articles 2 and 28 in relation to the quality of medical care,

5. This situation began to change with the accession of Assemblyman Alan Hevesi, an activist, to the Chairmanship of the Assembly Health Committee in 1977.

we must say that the record is spotty. Virtually nothing has been done in hospital ambulatory care. There has been activity in short-term hospital inpatient services and in long-term care, but that activity remains essentially unevaluated objectively, except for one study of certification-of-need. The powers of the department are plentiful. The legal sanctions are strong. Implementation has been, at best, inconsistent. The contrast between this inaction at the state level and what happened under the Ambulatory Care Program of the New York City Health Department is quite striking, and it is to a consideration of the ACP and Ghetto Medicine which we shall now turn.

References

Bernstein, G. Interview. North Woodmere, N.Y. Mar. 10, 1975.

Bicknell, W. J., & Walsh, D.C. Certification-of-need: The Massachusetts experience. *New England Journal of Medicine,* 1975, *292,* 1054.

Chapter 326, Laws of 1963. New York State Public Health Laws, Sec. 206 (1) (j).

Cicero, F. Interview. Albany, N.Y., May 13, 1975.

Cohen, H. S. Regulating health care facilities: The certificate-of-need process re-examined. *Inquiry,* 1973. *10,* 3.

Comptroller General of the United States. *Study of health facilities construction costs.* U.S. Government Printing Office. Washington, D.C., 1972.

Consumer Commission on the Accreditation of Health Services. Hospital inspection: Its importance to the consumer. *Health Perspectives,* 1974, *1,* Sept.–Oct. (a)

Consumer Commission on the Accreditation of Health Services. *Quarterly.* New York, N.Y., Winter 1974. (b)

Dorsey, J. L. Certification of need laws. *Archives of Surgery,* 1973, *10,* 765.

Fleck, A. Interview. Albany, N.Y., Mar. 7, 1975.

Folsom, M. B., et al. *Report of the Governor's committee on hospital costs.* New York, N.Y., 1965.

Garry, J. Interview. Albany, N.Y., May 13, 1975.

Hammerling, A. Interview. New York, N.Y., Apr. 2, 1975.

Havighurst, C. C. Regulation of health facilities and services by "Certificate of Need." *Virginia Law Review,* 1973, *59,* 1143.

Havighurst, C. C. Regulation in the health care system. *Hospitals*, J.A.H.A. *48*, June 16, 1974, p. 65. (a)

Havighurst, C. C. *Regulating health facilities construction*. American Enterprise Institute for Public Policy Research. Washington, D.C., 1974. (b)

Ingraham, H. S. Hospital affairs: New mission for the state health department. *New York State Journal of Medicine*, Mar. 15, 1966, p. 771.

Ingraham, H. S. *The Article 28 story: Landmark in health facility planning*. New York State Department of Health, Albany, N.Y., 1973.

Joint Legislative Committee on the Problems of Public Health, Medicare, Medicaid and Compulsory Health and Hospital Insurance. *Annual report: Legislative document No. 40*. Albany, N.Y., 1967.

Joint Legislative Committee on the Problems of Public Health, Medicare, Medicaid and Compulsory Health and Hospital Insurance. *Annual report: Legislative document No. 14*. Albany, N.Y., 1968.

Joint Legislative Committee on the Problems of Public Health, Medicare, Medicaid and Compulsory Health and Hospital Insurance. *Annual Report: Legislative document No. 19*. Albany, N.Y., 1969.

Joint Legislative Committee on the Problems of Public Health, Medicare, Medicaid and Compulsory Health and Hospital Insurance. *Annual report: Legislative document No. 8*. Albany, N.Y., 1970.

Leavy, W. *The Article 28 story: New York State's national leadership in health facility planning*. 1972. Process. Cited by Rathenberg (1975), p. 48.

McKinney's consolidated laws of the State of New York. St. Paul, Minn. See also "Pocket Parts."

Miller, H. Interview. Queens, N.Y., Apr. 10, 1975.

Morris Associates. *Health systems*. Washington, D.C., March 17, 1975, p. 3.

New York State Department of Health. *Our mission: Your health. Annual report, 1969*. Albany, N.Y., May, 1970.

New York State Department of Health. Decade of legislation. Oct. 13, 1971. Process.

New York State Department of Health. *New York State's health: Annual report, 1971*. Albany, N.Y., May, 1972.

New York State Department of Health. *New York State's health: Annual report, 1972*. Albany, N.Y., Apr., 1973.

New York State Department of Health. *Hospital program manual: Policy. Surveys: Article 28 surveys*. Item 821. Albany, N.Y., Aug. 3, 1973.

New York State Department of Health. *Annual report, 1973*. Apr. 1974.

O'Donoghue, D., et al. *Evidence about the effects of health care regulation: An evaluation and synthesis of policy relevant research.* Spectrum Research, Inc. Denver, Colo., 1974.

Official compilation codes, rules and regulations of the State of New York. 10 Health (A, B, and C). New York State, Albany, N.Y.

Pomrinse, S. D. Interview. April 4, 1975.

Reichman, S. Interview. New York, N.Y., April 4, 1975.

Rothenberg, E. *Evaluating the impact of certificate of need on hospital and health facilities planning outcomes: The New York State experience.* Doctoral Dissertation. New York University. New York, N.Y., June 1975. Process.

Rothenberg, E. *Regulation and Expansion of Health Facilities: The Certificate of Need Experience in New York State.* Praeger. New York, 1976.

Senate Finance Committee and Assembly Ways and Means Committee. *Hearings.* Albany, N.Y., Feb. 9, 1970.

Senate Finance Committee and Assembly Ways and Means Committee. *Hearings.* Albany, N.Y., Mar. 2, 1971.

Senate Finance Committee and Assembly Ways and Means Committee. *Hearings.* Albany, N.Y., Feb. 12, 1974.

Solomon, D. Interview. Albany, N.Y., May 13, 1975.

Task Force on Health: Report to Governor Carey. *New York State Department of Health: Major programs and responsibilities.* Albany, N.Y., December 1974.

Tenney, J. B., et al. National ambulatory medical care survey: Background and methodology. *Vital and Health Statistics.* Series 2, No. 61, 1974.

37 nursing homes face state fines. *New York Times,* June 4, 1975.

Wainfeld, B. Interview. Brooklyn, N.Y., March 26, 1975.

Winslow, C.-E. A. *The life of Herman M. Biggs.* Lea & Febiger. Philadelphia, Pa., 1929.

Winslow, C.-E. A. The untilled fields of public health. *Science,* 1920, *51*, 23. Quoted in Winslow's *Life of Biggs,* p. 345.

5

The Historical Development
of Ghetto Medicine and
the Ambulatory Care Program

Historical Background

HERMAN BIGGS AND THE PROTOTYPE FOR HEALTH DEPARTMENT
ACTIVITY IN GENERAL MEDICAL CARE

The genesis of the Ghetto Medicine program can be found in the
Annual Report for 1919 of Herman Biggs, then Commissioner of
Health for the State of New York.[1] The report, delivered in April
1920, noted the severe problems which many rural communities
were having in obtaining medical service. It is indeed fascinating
to read Biggs's discussion of the problem of the maldistribution of
medical manpower and the reasons therefor, quoted at length by
Winslow and Terris. Biggs's statement could have been written today. To deal with the problem, Biggs proposed legislation to encourage the establishment throughout the state of local health
centers to house school medical, public health nursing, and public
health education services, to coordinate all existing rural public
health activities for tuberculosis, venereal disease, maternal and
child health, and the like, to provide laboratory and X-ray services,
and to also provide general medical services, both outpatient and
inpatient, on a sliding-fee scale, or free, if necessary. Biggs's memorandum describing the original bill is reproduced in Appendix 5.

---

1. The material for this section comes primarily from C.-E. A. Winslow's
Life of Herman M. Biggs, Lea & Febiger, Philadelphia, 1929, chap. 17; and
Milton Terris's "Herman Biggs' Contribution to the Modern Concept of the
Health Center," *Bulletin of the History of Medicine,* 1946, *20,* 387.

The proposal was, of course, a radical one. It would have established a group of government-operated comprehensive health-care centers providing a complete range of preventive and curative services. It ran into strong opposition from the State Medical Society. It was defeated the first time it was introduced, in the legislative session of 1920. It was reintroduced in 1921, and Biggs tried hard to deal with the medical profession. In a speech to the New York County Medical Society, he pointed out the advantages to rural practitioners of having laboratory and X-ray services available, of having colleagues to communicate with. He discussed the shortages of hospital beds in the rural areas, which the program would alleviate (shades of Hill-Burton!). He recalled earlier, fruitless, and groundless struggles on the part of the medical societies against venereal disease and tuberculosis reporting, saying, in effect, "You were wrong then and have admitted it, so why not see the error of your ways now?" He appealed to reason, to politics. Nothing worked. The opposition from the profession continued.

How familiar do the arguments of the opposition sound? The program would give "too much power to the laity and too little to the medical profession." It would be "a step toward centralization of government and paternalism," "a measure which, to a great extent tends to or does deprive us of our liberties." "It is an entering wedge toward state medicine; . . . it puts a large number of medical men on a salary, and so does away with, or deprives them of, initiative and individualism and must to a certain extent in that way lower the morale of the medical profession." Finally, the arguments went, a doctor associated with a health center would have an unfair advantage over a doctor not associated. The bill again was defeated.

In 1923, the program was reintroduced in the legislature, but in a different guise. There was no grand statement of purpose attached to the bill. It appeared simply in the form of a measure to provide for state aid to rural counties for "the construction, establishment or maintenance by such county of a county, community, or other public hospital, clinic dispensary or similar institution, or for the purpose of defraying the expenses of such county in any public enterprise or activity for the improvement of the public health." The term *health center* never appeared. The bill quietly passed this time, and became Chapter 662, Laws of 1923. However, at the moment of one of Biggs's greatest triumphs, realizing in law the principle that the separation between "preventive medicine" and "treatment medicine" is an entirely artificial one, that there is no logical reason for dividing "public health" from "medical care," gaining recognition of the fact that government responsibilities for health care for all of the people, poor or not, cannot be kept away from the bedside by some arbitrary line, Biggs died, on June 28, 1923, at the age of sixty-three.

The program was apparently never implemented, whether because of Biggs's death or for other reasons. But it does stand on the statute books as a landmark of progressive health care thinking. To this day no state has ever implemented a program of the type contemplated by Biggs, not even, as we shall see, New York with the passage of Ghetto Medicine 45 years later. Indeed, there is no country in the world, with the exception of Sweden and, in a few isolated instances, Japan, which has created a combined inpatient/outpatient, preventive/treatment health care institution of the type envisoned by Biggs.

LEGISLATIVE HISTORY OF THE PRESENT PROGRAM

In 1967, the New York State Department of Health decided to make another try at implementing Herman Biggs's idea of involving health departments directly in the delivery of general medical services.[2] The department was concerned about health care shortages in the rural areas of the state, as was Biggs, but it was also concerned about the increasing health care deficits in the so-called ghetto areas of high minority group population concentrations. Fleck prepared a short prospectus for the proposed program in June 1967. The general idea was to pass legislation enabling local departments to establish general medical clinics (which they could not do previously), to charge for services provided in them (going against the tradition of free-to-all-at-the-time-of-use Health Department services), and to waive the fees if departments chose to do so. The

2. Most of the legislative history of Ghetto Medicine came from the interview with Dr. Andrew Fleck on March 7, 1975, cited in chapter 4, and from unpublished documents supplied by him. Other material was also used, as noted.

programs envisioned would in fact have been financed for the most part by the state's then broad-coverage Medicaid program. It was estimated that about 90 percent of persons using such centers in the neighborhoods in which they would presumably be established would be Medicaid-eligible.

The legislative proposals were prepared in the fall of 1967 and introduced in the legislature in 1968. Interestingly, nowhere can one find a bill that has the label Ghetto Medicine on it. Further, nowhere can one find a bill which describes the program which the Health Department, and the state administration, of course, had in mind. The program was in fact created by two *separate* bills, each of which contained very brief amendments to the Public Health Law. Groundwork had been done with the Medical Society of the State of New York (MSSNY). Its approval was obtained, primarily because the programs were intended for under-doctored areas, and the Medical Society was very concerned at the time with Governor Nelson Rockefeller's proposal for a New York State Universal Health Insurance Program. The label Ghetto Medicine was invented by Fleck as part of his program to deal with MSSNY anxieties.

The two-bill approach was also part of the strategy of doing nothing to awaken opposition. On June 5, 1968, Chapter 572 of the New York State Laws of that year was passed without debate. This chapter amended the Public Health Laws to allow health commissioners in the several local jurisdictions to waive or compromise the collection of fees. At that time, commissioners could charge only for nursing and paramedical services in the home. In fact, these amendments had nothing to do with a change in departmental policy on home nursing services but were preparing the way for another series of amendments to come.

On June 17, 1968, Governor Rockefeller announced a three-part program for improving health care delivery in low-income urban and rural areas, including mobile detection units, "neighborhood health facilities," and a neighborhood health worker program. The proposal for neighborhood health facilities was buried in much verbiage about the other components of the program, and a great deal of emphasis was given to the maternal and child health aspects of the neighborhood health facilities part of the proposal.

On June 22, 1968, Chapter 967 of the Laws of 1968 passed the legislature without debate. Chapter 967 amended the Public Health Laws to allow the health commissioners in the various local government jurisdictions to establish general medical services and charge for such services. The State Health Department was careful to make sure that the program would be implemented through local health departments. The State Budget Division required this approach to make certain that the State Health Department would not get into the direct care business itself and thus possibly get into an open-ended spending situation. The charge-for-services feature was necessary if the centers were to be able to collect Medicaid reimbursement. The federal Medicaid legislation provides that institutions cannot bill for services to Medicaid-eligible persons which are given to non-Medicaid-eligible persons free of charge.

Chapter 967 was accompanied by a brief statement from the governor outlining its true purposes. Both chapters came up late in the legislative session, and because of Biggs's negative experience with public hearings, none were held. Avoidance of public discussion was part of the strategy. Thus was Ghetto Medicine established.

In 1969, modification was made with Chapter 35, Laws of that year, which allowed the health commissioners of the various jurisdictions to institute sliding-fee scales.

THE REGULATIONS, FUNDING, AND EARLY ATTEMPTS
TO IMPLEMENT THE PROGRAM

Regulations were written to implement the program. They consist of Health Code sections 40.10 (a) (2), 40.10 (c) (2), Part 703, and Section 39.3 (d). They are reproduced in part in Appendixes 6, 7, and 8. Somewhat more detailed regulations appear in the *State Aid Manual*, not a formalized code of any sort but the State Health Department's day-to-day working guide book.

In brief, the code provides: Ghetto Medicine clinics have to be approved by the Department of Health; Subchapter F of the State Hospital Code, which pertains to free-standing ambulatory care units, is to be complied with; there is a fee schedule; the local health commissioner is allowed to waive collection of fees; the local health commissioner is to have general supervisory control; services may be provided under contract; there must be a community advisory committee; and state formula aid will be available to cover up to 50 percent of expenses not otherwise reimbursed.

The state aid formula for the Ghetto Medicine program is the traditional one for local government categorical public health programs. The state provides 50 percent of the cost of approved local government categorical services, and it continued this approach for Ghetto Medicine. It was assumed, of course, that since most patients using services would be Medicaid-eligible, the unreimbursed part of the cost would be low, and that a 50/50 sharing approach would put an undue burden on neither the state nor the local government jurisdictions. This is the origin of the "deficit-funding" character of the Ghetto Medicine which was carried into its later transformation to a hospital-subsidy program in New York City. In 1967, Fleck estimated that the direct cost to the state (exclusive of the state's share of the Medicaid expenditures, of course), would be $500,000 for a statewide program providing one million visits in 1968, growing to $4,725,000 for a seven-million-visit program in 1971. The clinic visit rates which he projected were $10.00 for 1968 and $13.50 for 1971.

Early approaches to implementation of Ghetto Medicine were undertaken in New York City. During 1969, negotiations between the state, the city, and three voluntary hospitals led to three contracts for the provision by the voluntaries of general medical services in three New York City Health Department District Health Centers, one of which had been previously funded entirely by the city (McLaughlin et al., 1971). Although not exactly what had been originally conceived of, since it was not the Health Department which was undertaking the program itself, but a voluntary hospital under contract, at least general medical services were being provided from Health Department District Health Centers which had previously provided only traditional categorical services. However, the development of programs of this type in New York City was overtaken by other health care events which would lead to previously undreamed of changes in the direction of the entire program.

Outside of New York City, Ghetto Medicine programs were developed in six counties: Albany, Erie, Westchester, Monroe, Nassau, and Suffolk. In chapter 7, Suffolk County is considered in detail. We were unable to find any State Health Department summary reports on Ghetto Medicine, either excluding or including New York City. Nor does any mention of Ghetto Medicine appear in the Department's Annual Reports for 1969 and 1971–73 (New York State Department of Health 1970, 1972-74). Total state expenditures for Ghetto Medicine outside of New York City for 1972–75 were: 1972, $834,732; 1973, $998,396; 1974, $1,622,221; 1975 (est.), $2,172,530. Thus as we shall see, the major action took place in New York City.

Ghetto Medicine in New York City

ORIGINS

In the 1968 state legislative session, the same one which passed Ghetto Medicine without debate, major cutbacks were made in the state's Medicaid Program. These cuts, made in April 1968, took the heart out of the Ghetto Medicine program, which was to have been funded largely by Medicaid, before it could even be started. Oddly enough, no one seemed to realize at the time what the implications of the Medicaid cuts really were the Ghetto Medicine program. Perhaps if someone had, the proposal would have been withdrawn. The cuts reduced the Medicaid maximum annual income eligibility level for a family of four from $6,000 to $5,300 and removed from eligibility all persons between 21 and 64 who were not on welfare.

The comprehensive care program as originally conceived was thus crippled. In fact, in the summer of 1968, a meeting of State Senator Norman Lent's Joint Legislative Committee on Problems of Public Health, Medicare, Medicaid, and Compulsory Health and Hospital Insurance, attended by the senior State Health Department staff, was held to consider how the Ghetto Medicine program might be used by localities to deal with problems created by the Medicaid cutbacks. This was an exact reversal of the original approach, which had been to build the Ghetto Medicine program on a Medicaid base! In New York City, the Health Department did stubbornly push ahead with its contract idea determined to try to implement the Ghetto Medicine concept even with reduced support from Medicaid.

In 1969, two more significant events occurred. The Medicaid maximum annual income eligibility level was further reduced, to $5,000 for a family of four, and a state freeze on Medicaid reimbursement rates to hospitals was put into effect. The two consecutive cutbacks and the freeze threw the voluntary hospitals of New York City, which provide about 50 percent of all hospital clinic visits in the city, into an uproar. They faced mounting deficits in their ambulatory service operations with no prospect of a way out.

In the fall of 1969, the voluntary hospitals brought an increasing amount of pressure to bear on Governor Rockefeller. The state administration wanted to do something to help but did not want to have to pass new laws, which would have required calling the state legislature back into session. Casting about for an existing piece of legislation under which help could be provided, they discovered Ghetto Medicine as a vehicle. The Health Code section written pursuant to Chapter 967, L. 1968, Section 40.10 (c) (2) (ii) (f), did allow for the provision of services by contract (App. 6). Thus, by using a great deal of imagination, the way was left open for the City Health Department to contract with voluntary hospitals for the provision of ambulatory services, even if there did happen to be existing services in existing clinics. Governor Rockefeller found $6 million and made his move. At the same time, he speeded up advance payments against hospital Medicaid billings, for all services, on a temporary basis. Thus a whole new chapter in the development of the health care delivery system in the United States was begun without the addition of even one new chapter to the laws of the state in which the new beginning was made.

ORIGINAL CHARACTERISTICS OF THE NEW YORK CITY
AMBULATORY CARE PROGRAM

The New York City Health Department moved rapidly to implement the new form, the Ghetto Medicine program.[3] It came to be called officially the New York City Ambulatory Care Program (ACP), the term which we shall use, but many persons still call it Ghetto Medicine. A Bureau of Ambulatory Care was established in

3. This section is based on interviews with Gilbert Bernstein (1975), Andrew Fleck (1975), Stanley Reichman (1975), Al Schwarz (1975), and Benjamin Wainfeld (1975), and on the paper by McLaughlin et al. (1971).

the Health Department. The bureau's first director was Gilbert Bernstein, then an assistant commissioner in the department. Ground rules were quickly established. The money would be given to the hospitals by contract, since that was a mechanism which was already provided for in the Health Code, Section 40.10 (c) (2) (ii) (f). Since the state funding approach in the original Ghetto Medicine program had been to provide direct support for program deficits incurred after all third-party payments, principally Medicaid, had been collected—that is, deficit funding—the approach was continued in the voluntary hospital subsidy program.

Technically, the City Health Department would contract to pay for part of the deficits incurred by the voluntaries in their ambulatory services operations, and then collect a portion of that payment from the state. The traditional state aid formula was to be used for this program, that is, reimbursement of 50 percent of approved city expenditures. Thus in effect, the state would match city expenditures on a dollar-for-dollar basis up to the limit of the state appropriation for each given fiscal year. The city decided to use a 50%-of-deficit formula in setting the funding levels to be used in dealing with the voluntaries.

According to Fleck, there was nothing in the law or the code requiring the City Health Department to choose this level. They could have picked 100 percent or 23.8 percent or any other figure just as readily. This level was apparently just a simple, arbitrary, transfer from the state's 50%-aid-to-localities figure. In fact, according to Al Schwarz, Assistant Commissioner in the City Health Department and Director of the ACP in 1975, the payments to hospitals over the years never reached a level of covering 50 percent of deficits because of shortages of total funds available and the city's desire to provide at least some financial assistance to as many hospitals as possible under the program (1975).

With the basic guidelines and policies contained in Section 40.10 (c) (2) (ii) of the Health Code (Appendix 6) in hand, the City Health Department proceeded to negotiate contracts with the voluntary hospitals (McLaughlin et al.). The first contracts covered the period December 1969 through June 1970. Many of them were written and signed after the contract period began. Payments were made retroactively. Twenty-nine hospitals applied for funds and, for twenty-two of them, contracts were negotiated and signed. The total outlay was about $9.5 million. The participation by hospital, with the amount of money contracted for, by contract period through June 30, 1975, is shown in Table 5–1.

Many policies and precedents were set during the incredibly hectic first seven months of the program's existence. Although by law three parties were involved in each contract negotiation—the State Department of Health, the City Department of Health, and the hospital—the latter two were the major participants, with the state playing an approval role only. Within the City Health Department, there were divergent views of how the program should be implemented. The first meeting between City Health Department officials and hospital representatives was held at Bellevue Hospital late in 1969 (Bernstein, 1975). Commissioner Mary McLaughlin said, in effect; "We want you to come in. There will not be many regulations. We will not enforce them severely." Assistant Commissioner Gilbert Bernstein took a contrasting position. He said, in effect: "We will throw a lasso out, surrounding a pot of money. If you step inside to get the money, we will begin to draw in the lasso. You will be forced to change and, as time goes on, and money becomes tougher to get, you will have to change more." History has shown that Bernstein's approach prevailed.

The major provisions of the first series of contracts negotiated between the hospitals and the City Health Department for the December 1, 1969–June 30, 1970, period were as follows, in summary:

1. Services provided by the hospital's clinics were to be "comprehensive" and "family-oriented."
2. The Commissioner of Health was to have general supervision over the program.
3. The hospital was to provide all resources necessary to provide a broadly comprehensive set of specified services.
4. There was to be a Director of the Ambulatory Care Unit who had to meet certain standards and whose appointment had to be approved by the City Health Commissioner.
5. There had to be an Ambulatory Care Advisory Committee.
6. Preference in future employment had to be given to per-

sons residing in "economically deprived areas served by the Unit."

7. An appointment system was required.
8. The unrestricted right of inspection was given to the City Health Commissioner or his/her designee, and operation reports must be made available at the request of the Commissioner.
9. Patients referred from the ambulatory service to the hospital itself for admission had to be admitted and treated under the same rules as were applied to any other admittees.
10. The hospital was specifically constrained from reducing total volume of service. There had to be a maintenance of effort at the same time services are being improved. In fact, the hospital were specifically prohibited from using the money for new services, except as specified in the contract, but had to use the funds to maintain and improve existing services.
11. All Medicaid eligibility and collection responsibilities lay with the hospital.
12. Termination was allowed upon 30 days notice.
13. A fee schedule was required.

In the context of the manner in which most government funds were, and are, given to voluntary hospitals, these provisions were truly revolutionary. For the first time, funds were paid to hospitals for services *in the hospital* by contract. Standards of care were established for contracting hospital ambulatory care services. Fees and charges were standardized. Community participation, particularly in relation to contract enforcement, regulation, and inspection, was accepted by the hospitals. At the same time, they committed themselves to program improvements while maintaining their previous level of effort. At first called "guidelines," detailed regulations were written pursuant to the prototype contract. The first written draft of those guidelines did not appear until a year later, in the spring of 1971. It is reproduced in Appendix 9. The interested reader will want to compare them with their 1975 descendants, the Contract Schedules, which are reproduced in part in Appendix 10. A consideration of the experience of the first 15 months of the pro-

TABLE 5-1

Expenditures for Ambulatory Care Program in New York City by Hospital, December 1969–June 1975

Hospital	12/1/69–6/30/70	7/1/70–6/30/71	7/1/71–6/30/72	7/1/72–6/30/73	7/1/73–6/30/74	7/1/74–6/30/75
Beekman Downtown	—	—	—	200,000	263,000	277,500
Beth Israel	1,706,700	3,765,600	332,400	288,200	360,000	379,800
Bronx Lebanon	869,000	1,650,000	1,050,000	945,000	1,145,000	1,208,000
Brookdale	349,400	751,200	665,000	665,700	764,300	806,300
Brooklyn	—	—	—	152,800	211,100	222,700
Columbus	202,300	391,200	293,300	240,200	327,200	345,200
French & Polyclinic	288,800	351,000	350,600	398,800	250,000	400,000
Joint Diseases	367,300	855,600	605,500	708,600	822,500	867,700
Jamaica	259,100	194,600	—	41,700	150,000	158,300
Jewish of Brooklyn	119,800	—	—	92,700	179,100	188,900
Jewish Memorial	—	—	—	—	80,000	168,800
Kingsbrook Jewish	—	—	—	—	100,000	211,000
Knickerbocker-Logan	292,800	235,200	192,000	580,000	1,012,000	611,900

Lutheran of Brooklyn	—	—	—	—	50,000	105,500
Lutheran Medical Center	102,400	300,000	193,000	143,200	200,500	211,500
Maimonides	—	—	—	364,200	443,600	468,000
Mary Immaculate	340,000	476,400	283,100	416,700	501,400	529,000
Methodist	260,400	277,200	303,900	259,900	383,900	405,000
Misericordia	219,200	561,600	314,700	301,100	374,200	394,800
Montefiore	548,200	615,000	1,055,200	994,100	1,136,500	1,199,000
Mt. Sinai	683,500	1,065,000	1,589,600	1,428,500	1,614,300	1,703,000
Flower & Fifth	70,300	213,600	191,800	93,800	146,200	154,200
NENA[a]	—	—	—	64,700	100,000	105,500
Roosevelt	360,900	1,282,500	1,105,300	676,600	787,300	830,600
St. Clare's	219,400	386,400	234,600	278,200	349,000	368,200
St. John's	219,700	140,400	228,000	182,300	243,500	256,900
St. Luke's	496,100	241,500	848,500	822,200	947,400	999,500
St. Mary's	335,000	572,400	152,900	231,100	347,200	366,300
St. Vincent's N.Y.	776,300	1,555,800	1,200,000	1,058,400	1,207,300	1,273,600
St. Vincent's S.I.	—	57,300	136,700	123,300	154,100	162,600
Total	$9,475,000	$16,220,900	$12,446,100	$11,792,000	$14,218,500	$15,379,300

SOURCE: Consumer Commission on Accreditation of Health Services. *Health Perspectives*, 1975, Vol. 2, No. 1 (January—February). Used by permission.
[a]North East Neighborhood Association.

gram in some further detail is reported in the papers by McLaughlin et al. (1971) and Betty Bernstein (1972).

It is apparent that something new and different was launched in New York City in the winter of 1969–70, albeit in a rather haphazard, unplanned way. The next chapter will consider the ACP as it stood in a comparatively mature stage, in the spring of 1975.

References

Bernstein, B. What happened to "Ghetto Medicine" in New York State. *American Journal of Public Health. 61*, 1287, 1971. See also relevant letters, *AJPH*, 1972, *62*, 3.

Bernstein, G. Interview. North Woodmere, N.Y., Mar. 10, 1975.

McLaughlin, M. C. et al. Ghetto medicine: Program in New York City. *New York State Journal of Medicine.* Oct. 1, 1971, p. 2321.

New York City Health Department. *Agreement made and entered into as of the 1st day of December 1969.* New York, N.Y. Process.

New York State Department of Health. *Our mission: Your health. Annual report, 1969.* Albany, N.Y. May 1970.

New York State Department of Health. *New York State's health. Annual report, 1971.* Albany, N.Y. May 1972.

New York State Department of Health. *New York State's health. Annual report, 1972.* Albany, N.Y. April 1973.

New York State Department of Health. *Annual report, 1973.* Albany, N.Y. April 1974.

Schwarz, A. Interviews, New York, N.Y., Mar. 12 and Apr. 16, 1975, and subsequent telephone conversations.

6

New York City's Ambulatory Care Program in 1975

Introduction

By 1975, the ACP had been operating for about five years.[1] Thirty hospitals were participating, receiving over $15 million in aid (Table 5–1). The number of visits for participating hospitals during 1972 and 1974 are shown in Table 6–1. The amount of money expended and visit volume do not alone indicate the significance of a hospital's participation in the program. The United Hospital Fund has developed a ranking scheme for ACP hospitals which takes into account the volume of ambulatory visits and the ratios of visits to beds and admissions. The summary of that effort, which identifies the "ten leading ACP hospitals," is shown in Table 6–2.

The 1975 prototype ACP contract was similar to the first contract, described in chapter 5. The language was refined and some more detail was added. There was one major program addition, partial default. The "guidelines," however, underwent significant change and became critical in defining the character of the program. The guidelines were transformed into Schedules and now constitute a formal attachment to an integral part of the contract. Schedule A contains the provisions for, and detailed rights and duties of, the community advisory groups which became formally the Community Boards for Ambulatory Care. Schedule B contains prototypical com-

1. There were several significant changes in the funding sources, the inspection system, and the mode of allocation of funds to the several hospitals which took place during the year following the completion of our original study in May 1975. They are described in a separate section at the end of this chapter.

TABLE 6-1

Number of Visits, ACP Participating Hospitals, 1972–74

HOSPITALS	1972			1974		
	Clinics	Emergency Room	Total	Clinics	Emergency Room	Total
Beekman Downtown	21,199	28,674	49,873	27,582	34,238	61,820
Beth Israel	—	42,652	42,652	—	42,302	42,302
Bronx Lebanon	123,000	61,000	184,000	122,523	70,004	192,527
Brookdale	117,010	58,126	175,136	103,121	65,484	168,605
Brooklyn	20,949	20,780	41,729	16,702	19,375	36,077
Columbus	25,869	9,963	35,832	37,118	15,116	52,234
French & Polyclinic	55,133	35,299	90,432	—	—	—
Joint Diseases	77,525	31,161	108,686	72,050	24,690	196,740
Jewish of Brooklyn	107,874	43,689	151,563	—	—	—
Jewish Memorial Hospital	27,274	16,704	43,978	28,319	16,189	44,508
Jamaica	23,460	44,451	67,911	28,664	36,441	165,105
Kingsbrook Jewish Medical Ctr.	23,854	9,153	33,007	19,698	8,210	27,908

Knickerbocker-Logan Memorial	28,992	21,551	50,543	27,120	18,278	45,938
Lutheran Medical Center	75,929	38,216	114,145	101,710	34,402	136,112
Lutheran Hospital of Brooklyn	9,624	19,263	28,887	—	—	—
Maimonides	84,647	45,974	130,621	66,176	50,956	117,132
Mary Immaculate	42,074	38,873	80,947	56,287	36,920	93,207
Methodist	38,583	45,453	85,036	47,185	55,637	102,822
Misericordia	35,286	29,745	65,031	30,541	27,361	57,902
Montefiore	108,084	47,664	155,748	141,781	62,459	204,240
Mt. Sinai	204,337	66,912	271,249	215,187	58,828	274,015
New York Medical–Flower & Fifth	19,189	14,824	34,013	34,612	23,528	58,140
Roosevelt	179,635	52,145	231,780	195,670	50,893	246,563
St. Clare's	34,130	20,580	54,710	30,479	24,391	54,870
St. John's	51,950	38,919	90,869	58,484	38,706	97,190
St. Luke's	176,320	83,054	259,374	207,372	85,191	292,563
St. Mary's	63,228	41,729	104,957	74,744	35,689	110,433
St. Vincent's of N.Y.	87,172	40,677	127,849	70,665	41,529	111,594
St. Vincent's of Richmond	20,821	23,709	44,530	25,280	32,848	58,128

SOURCE: Bureau of Ambulatory Care, New York City Health Department.

TABLE 6–2

*The Ten Leading Ambulatory Care Program Hospitals
as Measured by Volume and Visits/Beds
and Visits/Admissions Ratios*

HOSPITAL	Volume (Visits)	Ratio Visits/Beds	Visits/Admissions
1. Roosevelt	3	1	1
2. Catholic Medical Center	4	2	1
3. St. Luke's	2	4	2
4. Mt. Sinai	1	7	4
5. Brookdale	6	5	5
6. Joint Diseases	8	6	3
7. St. John's Episcopal	10	3	6
8. St. Vincent's, New York	7	9	7
9. Methodist	9	8	8
10. Montefiore	5	10	9

SOURCE: United Hospital Fund. Workbook on Ambulatory Care. No date, but presumably 1975. Used by permission.

munity board bylaws. Schedule C contains specific contract requirements for individual hospitals, in addition to the general program requirements spelled out in the contract and accompanying schedules. Schedules D and E contain the detailed Outpatient Department and Emergency Room Guidelines, respectively. (A summary of Schedules D and E is reproduced in Appendix 10.) Schedules F and G are concerned with the Fee Schedule and administrative rules. Perusal of the contract and schedules shows that the requirements for participation placed upon the hospitals are very detailed and in certain respects rather stringent, confirming Gilbert Bernstein's prediction of what would happen to the lasso inside of which the money has been placed.

The payments to hospitals were related to the deficits which they suffer in their ambulatory care programs reported in City Health Department audited figures. However, because of shortage of funds, payments have never reached the 50-percent-of-deficit level provided by state law. In no year of the existence of Ghetto Medicine, however, has the city treasury matched the funds made available for the program by state appropriation. Since 1973, the state has provided certain funds which voluntary hospitals in the ACP may match with their own money raised through voluntary contributions.

The ACP as an entity is nowhere mentioned in the State Public Health Laws. It is maintained on a year-to-year basis by appropriation only. Likewise, the city has never enacted a local law embodying the ACP. Further, the very detailed city ACP regulations have never been incorporated into its own health code. The program is in fact probably of questionable legality, particularly when its origins are taken into account.

The State Health Department has maintained a general hands-off posture in relation to the ACP. Contracts apparently receive the legally required approval by the State Health Commissioner rather automatically. No City Health Department inspection team has ever been accompanied by a State Health Department representative. All of this means that the collective power which the two departments have has never been put together.

The Community Role in the ACP

A community role is mandated in the state regulations governing the Ghetto Medicine program.[2] It appears in the Health Code, Sections 40.10 (a) (2) and (c) (2) (App. 6 of this book). It also appeared in the provisions for Ghetto Medicine originally written into the *State Aid Manual*. According to several informants, including David Pomrinse (1975), the strong political pressure which had been brought to bear on Governor Rockefeller by interests in the city who were opposed to aiding the voluntary hospitals without at least also helping the municipal hospitals (something which was never done), was in part responsible for creating a strong community presence in the program. It was part of the package which the state administration put together to sell the program in the city.

2. Material for this section comes from papers by McLaughlin, et al. (1971), and B. Bernstein (1972), cited in chapter 5, and Bellin et al. (1972); interviews, cited in chap. 4, with A. Hammerling (1975), Dr. S. D. Pomrinse (1975), and Dr. B. Wainfeld (1975); in chapter 5 with A. Schwarz (1975); interviews with Zita Fearon (1976) and Gary Gambuti (1975); and interviews with other persons who did not wish to be quoted directly.

According to Lowell Bellin, City Health Commissioner in 1975, the voluntary hospitals were so desperate for money that they were ready to accept almost any conditions (1972).

Structure and Responsibilities. In 1975, the structure for community participation in the ACP was as follows (Consumer Commission, 1975; Fearon, 1976; McCann, 1974): For each hospital, as mandated by the ACP contract, there was a Community Board, originally called The Ambulatory Services Advisory Committee. Membership size ranged from 11 to 17, with an average membership of 15. The boards had both consumer and hospital representatives. The hospital's Director and the Director of Ambulatory Care had to be included among the latter. The local City Health Department District Health Officer sat on them as well. The boards all had a consumer majority, but, generally, consumers constituted no more than 60 percent of the board membership. It was intended that about one-half of the consumer representatives be patients who used the services themselves, with the balance representing community organizations. Any consumer member could serve a maximum of three one-year terms. The selection of the consumer members of the board was carried out in a variety of ways: nomination by consumer organizations, special elections, suggestions by the Health Department, self-nomination, and the like. There had to be at least eleven meetings per year, including at least three public meetings. Each board had its own annual budget of $2,000, supplied by the City Health Department.

By 1971, there was a citywide steering committee of Ambulatory Care Community Board representatives. This evolved into the Consumer Council to the New York City Health Department, also referred to as the Ambulatory Care Consumer Advisory Committee. It met with City Health Department officials on a monthly basis to discuss problems and prospects of the ACP as a whole. In 1975, it had 30–40 members representing all of the Community Boards plus several citywide health consumer organizations. Like each Community Board, the Consumer Council had an annual budget of $2,000, supplied by the City Health Department.

The rights and scope of work of the Community Boards are spelled out in Schedule A of the contract (1974, p. 2–A). In brief the rights are as follows:

1. The right to full discussion of issues deemed important by the Board.
2. The right to consult with responsible officials and outside authorities.
3. The right to make specific recommendations to responsible officials.
4. The right to health education programs for the community.
5. The right to inspect the ambulatory services based on a plan presented to and approved by the Commissioner of Health.
6. The right to be involved in the early stages of planning and the right to be consulted within adequate time about policies affecting Ambulatory Care.

The Community Boards are to "advise and consult" with the Hospital and the City Health Department on the following items: (1) Quality of care, (2) Physical plant standards, (3) Maintenance of facilities, (4) Patient registration, (5) Patient eligibility, (6) Fee schedules, (7) Billing for self-pay patients, (8) Staffing patterns, (9) Establishment of health priorities, (10) Hours of service, (11) Review and follow-up of patient grievances, (12) Methods of handling patient admissions from outpatient department, (13) Complying with the terms of the contract. In addition (14), all reports are to be made available to the Community Board; (15) a patients' rights document consistent with the general aims of the agreement was to be developed; and (16) the Community Board may use the site-visit report and information available from patients to measure the compliance of the hospital with major items in the body of the contract, e.g., comprehensiveness of care, primary physician care, supervision, and involvement of the Community Board in hospital decisions.

Evaluation of Performance. As might be expected, the quality of performance of the Community Boards varies. No objective evaluation of Community Board functioning has ever been carried out. An authoritative source who represents consumer interests in the city said that the criteria for good functioning should include at least: (1) an active, consistent consumer membership; (2) ability to communicate with the hospital and the City Health Department on problems; (3) the ability to get goal-oriented practical projects for improving ambulatory services underway with active Community Board participation; (4) the ability to maintain a constructively critical relationship with the hospital, becoming neither nonproductively negative toward nor noncritically protective of the hospital.

According to these criteria, in 1975 the "best" boards were described as the ones at Brookdale, Lutheran Medical Center, Maimonides, Methodist, Roosevelt, St. Luke's, and St. Vincent's. The "worst" boards were considered to be at Beekman-Downtown, Catholic Medical Center, Montefiore, Brooklyn Hospital, and Mount Sinai. This view was generally concurred in by other observers queried. "Co-opted" was the appellation generally given to the Community Boards considered "worst." This view, which may or may not be valid, considers that if a board spends a great deal of time defending "its" hospital to the City Department of Health and its inspectors, it is not doing its job properly.

An analysis in detail of Community Board functioning was not within the purview of this study. A doctoral dissertation on the subject has been written (Metsch, 1972). Major features of the study have been summarized (Metsch & Veney, 1974). The study director did have the opportunity to attend a meeting of one Community Board which is generally considered to be "co-opted" by citywide consumer representatives. The meeting was instructive in several ways. The chairman of the board was a member of the hospital administration. This is permitted under the guidelines for bylaws, but it is unusual. The group did spend a great deal of time either in procedural wrangling or general philosophical discussion. Thus it had little time or energy left to become concerned with substance specific to the hospital, or with the development of projects to improve services with which the board could possibly become involved. All consumer representatives who spoke up voiced at least as many criticisms of the Health Department as they did of the hospital. Nevertheless, one consumer/patient member of the board interviewed briefly after the meeting did feel that the board has been effective and has brought about improvements in service.

Of special interest at this meeting was that the first substantive statement by a consumer representative concerned problems on the inpatient service rather than the outpatient service. The hospital representatives eventually turned the discussion aside by continually reiterating that the purview of the board did not extend to the inpatient side and that the patient should talk to the chairman of the appropriate medical staff committee. In an interview with the study director held just before the meeting, the director of the hospital had been very positive in his evaluation of the functioning of the Community Board. He had been asked whether, if the Community Board had played a valuable role in the improvement of ambulatory care, it would not be a good idea to create a community board with responsibilities for inpatient services as well. The first response was active recoil from the suggestion, followed by the position that there already was in existence a community board, the Board of Trustees. Finally the director said, referring to the consumer members of the board: "Well, those people aren't interested in inpatient services anyway."

The director of another hospital whose Community Board was characterized as "co-opted" described his hospital's board as "excellent, intelligent . . . understands our problems. Elsewhere," he said, "Boards are not so good. The Board has increased our understanding of patient views . . . but brought no major changes." Other hospital representatives representing hospitals whose Community Boards are considered "good" by citywide consumer representatives —that is, "tough" and not co-opted—had different views, however. Alden Hammerling of Roosevelt (1975, cited in chap. 4) considered that the board has "played a positive role," "keeps us on target," "adds momentum," and "reinforces our commitment." Gary Gambuti of St. Luke's said (1975): "They keep us on our toes. It's good. Things happen that might not happen or might take longer without them."

In sum, the community role in the ACP is one of contract enforcer. With some degree of variation, in 1975 the boards appeared to be active, and productive.

Evaluating Hospital Performance under the ACP

STANDARDS FOR EVALUATION

From the inception of the ACP, there have been performance standards which participating hospitals have been bound to meet under the contract. At first, they were contained in the contract itself, stated simply and briefly. As was noted above, the first program "guidelines" made their appearance in the spring of 1971 (App. 9). They dealt with such matters as the provision of primary care, the existence of a director of ambulatory care, inpatient admission procedures, an appointment system, interpretation services, laboratory standards, pharmacy, radiology, the creation of a procedures manual, physical plant, medical records, professional staffing, waiting time, drop-in clinics, evening clinics, clinic schedules, nutrition, types of medical services to be offered, staff training, quality audits and follow-up. As noted above, by 1975 the "guidelines" had become Schedules, formally incorporated into the contract.

The detailed service operating standards are contained in Schedules D and E, "Outpatient Department" and "Emergency Room" respectively. They cover the same ground as did the original 1971 guidelines, but they have grown from eight double-spaced, typewritten pages to twelve single-spaced pages. For example, where social work was dealt with by nine lines in 1971, the requirements now cover two single-spaced pages. In Appendix 10, Schedules D and E are briefly summarized.

CITY HEALTH DEPARTMENT EVALUATION PROCEDURES

The right and responsibility of the City Health Department to inspect and evaluate the performance of the ambulatory services in participating hospitals is an essential part of the contract. Hospitals were inspected by the department's Bureau of Ambulatory Care with a frequency of slightly more than one time per year. (In 1976, a reduction in the bureau's staff lead to a drop in the frequency of inspections.) Attempts were being made to provide for Community Board inspections, using a modified Health Department protocol. Such inspections could not themselves lead to sanctions against the hospital, but they could lead to the calling in of the Health Department to look at specific problems. The major features of the evaluation procedure in 1975 were as follows (Schwarz & Furman, 1975):

1. The site-visits are made by appointment. The hospitals are required to prepare information on utilization, staffing, scheduling, and the like in advance.

2. The site-visit team includes central office nonphysician and physician staff. Also invited are the Health Department's local District Health Officer and representatives of the Community Board.
3. The first event of the site-visit is a meeting between the site-visit chairperson (a City Health Department staffer) and the Community Board, during which the chairperson makes an attempt to evaluate the effectiveness of the board, and attempts to make sure that the board understands its rights under the contract.
4. The physician member of the team carries out medical chart review, using primarily process, and occasionally, outcome criteria.
5. The team directly observes clinic and emergency room activity, using both structural and process criteria for evaluation.
6. An exit interview sums up the day, with particular attention paid to the role of the Director of Ambulatory Care and the organization of the Clinics and the Emergency Room.
7. A report of the visit is submitted to the hospital within three weeks. Problems are detailed, and, if the department is planning to implement the partial default system, it is explained.

The standard follow-up procedure involves the exit interview session with the hospital's advisory board, attendance by Bureau of Ambulatory Care staff at the next advisory board meeting, at which time the report of the site-visit is explained (it is mailed out before this), a request to the hospital for a written timetable for implementation of necessary changes, and follow-up site-visits for continuing problems.

There are several central elements in the evaluation procedure. First, the Community Board is an integral part of it. Second, both structural and process measures of quality are used. There are many structural standards in Schedules D and E: types of clinics, hours of service, the requirement for an appointment system, the requirement for a Director of Ambulatory Care. However, unlike most other types of regulations for hospital operations, there are process standards as well: comprehensive, family-oriented primary care is to be provided, the delay in getting an initial appointment through the appointment system is not to exceed two weeks, the Director of Ambulatory Care shall have the authority to carry out his/her responsibilities. The evaluation thus examines not only whether or not a particular set of clinics exists, but also whether they are delivering a particular kind of product; not only whether an appointment system exists, but also whether it actually functions to a particular level; not only is there a Director of Ambulatory Care, but also does he/she actually have any power? Furthermore, there is the chart-review part of the evaluation which looks at the process of care in individual cases and may even consider outcomes of care in certain instances, at least insofar as outcomes may be represented in medical records. Third, inspections are not just done on a "one-shot" basis, but include written comments and, on occasion, follow-up visits.

Fourth, the inspections are related to payments. Beginning with the 1973–74 contracts, the Health Department took on the power to declare institutions in "partial default." Prior to 1974, it was an all-or-nothing proposition. If a hospital failed all or part of an inspection, the only possible penalty was dismissal from the program. Partial default, a much more sensitive tool, then became available. After review, part-payment could be withheld from a hospital with particular deficiencies until those deficiencies were corrected, without eliminating the hospital from the program entirely. This kind of approach means that hospitals can be assisted to improve, at the same time having a real incentive to improve. (In 1976, a complex "compliance formula" was introduced, relating the amount of payment to number of visits, size of deficit, and level of contract performance. It is discussed at the end of this chapter.)

STAFFING THE EVALUATION PROGRAM

The evaluation staff of the City Health Department's Bureau of Ambulatory Care is not limited, required, specified, or funded by any specific contract or agreement between the state of New York and the city of New York. The size and composition of the staff is purely a city decision, and funding is provided through the routine City/State, 50/50 mechanism used in "regular" City Health Department functions. In the spring of 1975, the staff consisted of:

1 full-time physician
1 full-time dentist
1 senior fiscal analyst
4 program research analysts
4 typists
1 clerk
1 administrative assistant
1 director
3 part-time medical specialist consultants
1 part-time administrative consultant

Until approximately one year before, there had been six more professional and three more clerical staff members. The reduction was due to city belt tightening. According to the Director of the Bureau of Ambulatory Care, one result of the cutbacks was that the Health Department visits became much more inspection-oriented than evaluation-oriented, a distinctly retrogressive event. Further staff cuts were made in 1976.

OUTCOMES OF EVALUATION

Hospital evaluation reports under the ACP are public documents. A comprehensive set of reports has been put together by the United Hospital Fund of New York (1975). Two reports, on Misericordia and Mount Sinai, were published by the Consumer Commission on the Accreditation of Health Services (January–February 1975).

Schwarz et al., in an unpublished work (June 1973), put together two prototypical case history/evaluation reports which are very illuminating for understanding how the evaluation system works and the results which it produces. It is reproduced in Appendix 11. The concluding paragraph is instructive:

> All too conclusively, the hospitals in the Ghetto Medicine Program offer stopgap, episodic care to too many persons in situations where comprehensive ambulatory care is called for both medically and in terms of the Ghetto Medicine Contract. Ghetto Medicine as it now stands is based on the premise that reorganization of the health system in New York City must start at the core of the voluntary sector, where the most power lies. A reorganization in this core is urgently needed. Ghetto Medicine can bring it about

only through a commitment to maximum pressure for comprehensive care and stringent enforcement of the mandates in the Ghetto Medicine Contract and Guidelines.

It is quite obvious that these evaluations, which are well worth reading, have breadth, depth, and real concern for the welfare of patients.

EVALUATIONS OF THE EVALUATIONS

It is no surprise that there is a wide range of opinion regarding the evaluation/inspection program and the City Health Department's approach to it. Gilbert Bernstein, the ACP's first director, and Al Schwarz, its director in 1975, generally regard the inspections as fair and productive, although they are always concerned with improving the procedures. Schwarz is very aware of the dangers inherent in government regulation of a too close relationship developing between regulator and regulatee (Schwarz et al., June 1973, p. 43). Lowell Bellin (1975), Commissioner of Health in 1975, First Deputy Commissioner of Health at the time of the inception of the ACP, felt that enforcement had become more strict, which he regarded as a positive event. Site-visits were being made more specific and more standardized, helpful for purposes of comparison. The reports were also being issued more quickly. Bellin was a strong supporter of the partial default system.

There are other views of the inspection/evaluations, of course. Gambuti (1975) felt that the site-visits were "terrible." He felt that the inspectors are "untrained and don't know what they are looking for." Much hospital staff time had to be spent responding to site-visit reports, which were, in Gambuti's words, "superficial," and contained "little new knowledge." He suggested in-depth evaluations of one specific outpatient department aspect or problem on each visit.

Hammerling (1975) felt that site-visits and reports were "positive, but too rigid." The hospital and the New York City program "share the same concerns." He saw the city as "a partner striving for common goals" and resented what he called their tendency to play "an adversary role," and "their lack of patience." The major problem was not with goals, but with feasible timing and with methods: "Methodological requirements are too rigid."

Another source felt that the Health Department had to be careful to avoid getting into a "checklist rut" in its approach to inspection/evaluation. The evaluators somehow have to become aware of day-to-day realities of the institutions which they are visiting. A second source, who did not wish to be quoted but who is known to be a strong supporter of consumer interests in health, characterized some Health Department recommendations as "absurd." He referred to the lack of continuity of inspectors. He felt that it is very difficult to make assessments in one day and that some major problems are missed. A Director of Ambulatory Care and an Associate Hospital Director characterized the inspectors as "arm-chair," "never on the firing line," "nonpractitioners," and, "worst of all [sic] nonphysicians." However, they also felt that ACP inspections could be used as levers for change.

Among the problems which exist in implementing the inspection/evaluation program in a positive way are the attitudes of the staff persons being evaluated. In another paper, Schwarz, with different colleagues, discusses this problem with particular reference to social service (Schwarz et al., November 1973).

Because the Ghetto Medicine Program reinforced the authority of the Department of Health, giving it the power to grant or withhold money to participating hospitals, resistance to the auditing process could be expected. Although the social service directors, as a group, were probably ahead of their hospital administrations in recognizing unmet needs of the outpatient department's clients, they resisted auditing as actively as did other hospital personnel. . . .

Although overt challenges to the judgment or authority of the health department were rare, there was covert or indirect resistance to evaluation on the part of the directors of social service. They were sometimes unprepared for site visits, even after having been given from one to two weeks' advance notice. Frequently, case records had not been assembled and statistics and other data requested in advance had not been compiled. One director was "out ill" on three site visits over a six-month period! . . .

Many of the covert messages received from the social service directors at meetings and in informal contact reflected their feelings of reproach and betrayal. Some of the directors felt that the department was somewhat unfair in exposing their short-comings. (After all, social workers should stick together against outsiders who do not understand the profession!) Some overt opposition emerged in reaction to the evaluation of productivity. . . .

The findings and conclusions of Schwarz et al., in reference to the attitudes of social workers to inspections, apply to other health professionals as well. If nothing else, inspections under the ACP shake people up, about themselves as well as about their building and their program.

Results of the Ambulatory Care Program

In our discussion of the implementation of Article 28 of the Public Health Laws of the State of New York and the codes written pursuant to it, we pointed out some of the immense, although not completely insoluble, difficulties confronting any attempts to objectively evaluate its results. How does one determine if the program has been implemented? How does one determine if codes are enforced? How does one determine what the effects of code enforcement are? Are the structural requirements which are found in most codes related to the quality of health care?

The same difficulties are to be faced in any attempt to evaluate the effects of the Ambulatory Care Program objectively. No comprehensive evaluation of the ACP has ever been carried out, and there is no ongoing evaluation system for it. Thus, as with the Article 28 program, no one really knows if the ACP made any difference insofar as the quality of care is concerned. Presumably, one tangible effect of the ACP has been to keep open outpatient departments in voluntary hospitals which otherwise, at least according to the hospitals themselves, would have been forced to close for financial reasons.

There was one small-scale attempt at objective evaluation of the ACP at one particular time, and there are, of course, many subjective evaluations which we encountered in the course of our interviews. In their 1973 report, Schwarz et al. examined the experience of twenty ACP hospitals in relation to seventeen program criteria, for the period Jan. 1, 1970–Jan. 1, 1973 (June 1973). The results are shown in Table 6–3. Most of the criteria are structural, but a few, like physician continuity, are process. For whatever it is worth, the experience shows progress on all but two measures

TABLE 6–3

Impact of the ACP on Seventeen Program Priorities

PRIORITY	Hospitals with Priority Item[a]			
	Jan. 1, 1970		Jan. 1, 1973	
	N	%	N	%
1. A full-time director of ambulatory care	12	60.0	17	85.0
2. A unit record system	14	70.0	17	85.0
3. Five or more sessions of medicine per week	11	55.0	15	75.0
4. Five or more sessions of pediatrics per week	7	35.0	10	50.0
5. Physician continuity	4	20.0	13	65.0
6. Ghetto medicine all inclusive sliding fee scale in the OPD	0	0.0	20	100.0
7. Professional review of diagnostic test results	10	50.0	18	90.0
8. Block or individual appointment system	7	35.0	11	55.0
9. Adult walk-in patients accommodated in the Outpatient Department	11	55.0	11	55.0
10. Pediatric walk-in patients accommodated in the Outpatient Department	9	45.0	12	60.0
11. OPD chart audit	6	30.0	15	75.0
12. ER chart audit	5	25.0	14	70.0
13. Triage in Emergency Room	2	10.0	4	20.0
14. Starter dose medications in the emergency room when Pharmacy closed	14	70.0	17	85.0
15. Physicians of resident level in the emergency room	18	90.0	18	90.0
16. Attending physician supervision of house staff in the Emergency Room	7	35.0	9	45.0
17. Ambulatory care services consumer advisory committee	0	0.0	20	100.0
Total	137	40.3	241	70.9

SOURCE: Schwarz, A., et al. "Evaluating Ambulatory Care in New York City." New York City Department of Health. Process. June 1973.
[a]Twenty-three hospitals participated in the program when it started in 1970. Three hospitals withdrew from the program due to inability to meet contract mandates.

(9 and 15), and compliance with criterion 15 was at a high level at the start of the program. Significant improvement in numbers of hospitals complying were found for physician continuity, institution of a sliding-fee scale, professional review of diagnostic test results, the institution of chart audits, and the establishment of a Consumer Board. This study, which has not been repeated, does not consider parameters of utilization, quality of medical care, or cost. It does, however, show that, on these criteria, the ACP had positive effects on the ambulatory services in the contracting hospitals.

Gilbert Bernstein (1975) felt that "things have changed and vastly improved" under the ACP. He pointed out that hospital inspections/evaluations naturally tend to concentrate on negatives rather than positives. Aside from the question of enforcement, the program established the same standards of care for all patients coming to the outpatient services, whereas before the ACP there were required standards only for Medicaid and Medicare patients. All patients presenting themselves had to be taken care of. The ACP has "put an end to intimidation and barriers to care created by Medicaid" with its means-test basis. At the same time, hospitals were required to "maintain their previous effort" in terms of volume of service. The ACP "pinned responsibility for in-patient care for patients coming to the out-patient department on the hospital as well." Fees and charges were standardized. Reports were made publicly available. Finally, Bernstein said, the participating hospitals accepted a few major changes in their modus operandi: community participation by persons from the lower socioeconomic class; the contract mechanism for obtaining operating funds; regulation and inspection by the City Department of Health.

Schwarz (1975) felt that the ACP had a "major impact." He agreed with Bernstein on the importance of the acceptance by the hospitals of the contractual obligation and consumer-participation. He pointed to the use of process standards in evaluation and felt that the program improved the quality of medical care in participating hospitals. Bellin (1975) also felt that the ACP improved the quality of medical care in ACP hospitals, if only because regular chart audits are a stimulus to improving the quality of medical records, which is itself related to the quality of medical care.

The Consumer Commission of the Accreditation of Health Services (January–February 1975) cited the following achievements: institution of the contract mechanism, particularly with the partial default system; the requirement for the provision of "dignified, comprehensive care"; the requirement for a director of ambulatory care; the institution of the sliding-fee schedule; the barring of the use of interns as primary physicians in the emergency room; the development of the Schedule C special requirements for each hospital.

Stanley Reichman (1975) agreed with most of the points made above. He also felt that the ACP was particularly important to his hospital, the Hospital for Joint Diseases. In several years its largest department, orthopedics, will be moving to the Beth Israel Medical Center and the rest of the institution will be converted into a general community hospital. On its Board of Trustees will likely be many people from the surrounding community. Thus, the ACP has provided an important learning experience for the institution in how to work with representatives of the working-class community.

Gambuti (1975) felt that overall the ACP had more positive than negative effects on hospitals. The impact on quality of care is difficult to assess, but the program, primarily through the presence of the Community Board, has improved the levels of dignity, comfort, convenience, and other factors closely related to patient satisfaction. He felt that the major defect in the ACP is that it only attacks details, and does not address basic problems or necessary organizational changes in ambulatory care. In fact, according to Gambuti, the ACP perpetuates the traditional patterns of outpatient department financing and staffing and does not require any alteration in the "stepchild" status of hospital ambulatory services. David Pomrinse (1975) thought that on the whole the ACP has been a good thing, but that its major impact was to "expedite changes which were already in the wind."

Benjamin Wainfeld (1975) of Brookdale saw improvements as a result of the ACP too. A particular feature at his hospital was a well-organized Grievance Committee of the Community Board. Wainfeld felt that this committee has been especially helpful in dealing with consumer-staff sensitivity sessions by the Community Board which appeared to lead to improved interpersonal relationships between staff and patients.

Illustrating the differences of opinion which exist within the hospitals themselves, at another institution the Hospital Director characterized the program as "the biggest farce ever perpetrated upon the public," while the Director of Ambulatory Care there considered it to be "very powerful in upgrading quality of care."

Zita Fearon (1975), Chairperson of the Council of Community Boards in 1975, was also enthusiastic about the program, citing many improvements noted by others. She cited the following as well: improved emergency room care, especially the removal of interns; the institution of appointment systems; the requirement for primary care physicians; the reduction in the number of specialty clinics; "slightly improved" patient care by doctors; patient-drug profiles being developed; increased emphasis on social service; nurse conferencing; the increasing of the awareness of health care issues on the part of many consumers. Lesser improvements were achieved in medical records, and Fearon reported, as did many others, that among the serious problems still remaining were those of the medical records systems: chart availability and accessibility, lack of completeness of entries, and missing lab and X-ray reports. Fearon would also like to see an ongoing evaluation of the functioning of the Community Boards, technical assistance to the boards themselves concerning substance and specific problem-solving, as opposed to emphasis on procedural problems.

Another consumer representative from a citywide group felt that the Ghetto Medicine program has improved the status of outpatient departments (OPDs). Consumer input to site-visits and hospital advisory boards has improved, although some consumer representatives "are manipulated" by hospitals. The availability of site-visit reports to the general public is a great step forward. In response to hospital allegations of methodological rigidity, it was felt that the current level of insistence on uniformity is necessary for reasonable assurance of progress. Exceptions are in fact made, and most hospitals have yet to achieve full compliance but continue to be paid. In the future more thorough control will be needed, according to this source, tied to the major sources of funding, not to a small supplement like the ACP. Hospitals will not act to improve quality of care or economy, or to meet patient needs, unless forced to do so.

Additional remaining problems cited by several observers include: many directors of ambulatory care have no control over physicians in the OPD; physician continuity is poor: resident rotations are brief, attendings are late and often absent; waiting times in scheduled clinics are too long (up to two hours); appointments for new patients take weeks, despite low patient/M.D. session ratios (often below three patients per M.D. hour); emergency rooms don't send patients back to original clinics for follow-up; record retrieval is poor: 20–30 percent of records are not found when needed, Emergency Room (ER) sheets are not included, preappointment record reviews are not done; there is poor follow-up of broken lab and X-ray appointments, and results are not posted quickly; many histories and physicals are incomplete; there is a lack of interpreters and multilingual signs. In summary, we do not have a broad-based objective assessment of the ACP, but we do have a remarkable agreement, for the most part, between hospital directors, directors of ambulatory care, City Health Department officials, and consumer representatives that the ACP has been a good thing and has achieved noticeable improvements in voluntary hospital ambulatory services in New York City.

Events in 1975–76

In the summer of 1975, the Select Committee on the Ambulatory Care Program, which included representatives from the participant hospitals, the City Health Department, and the Consumer Council to the New York City Health Department (the citywide coordinating group for the ACP Community Boards), promulgated a new formula for determining the amount of money which each receives under the ACP.[3] Previously it was related principally to the deficit incurred. Under the new formula, which was put into operation during the 1975–76 contract year, the amount of subsidy is related to the quality of the product delivered by the hospital in terms of compliance with the requirements of the contract and the patient load, as well as the size of the deficit.

3. This section is based upon interviews held with Robert Borsody, Zita Zearon, Al Schwarz, and Thomas Travers on July 12, 1976, and upon cited materials.

The formula is rather complex (New York City Health Department, May 1975). First, the degree of compliance by the hospital with the terms of its ACP contract is measured. The inspections have continued as before, but now there is a very detailed rating sheet which lists all of the contract requirements under about 45 main and 120 subsidy headings (NYC Health Department. 1975–76). Certain standards are made prerequisite for inclusion in the program. These include the requirement for a community board, its significant participation in hospital affairs, the requirement for a Director of Ambulatory Care, the prohibition against interns being primary staff in ambulatory services, and preferential hiring for local residents. The other standards are given weights, the total weights adding up to 100. The weights range from 0.1, for having clinic walk-in patients seen by their regular practitioner whenever possible, to 3.0 for having a medical audit committee for ambulatory services. If the hospital has complied with a particular standard, it receives the full weight allotted to the standard; if it has not complied, it receives nothing for that standard. Its total compliance, then, is additive and is a percentage.

Next, in determining the subsidy, the volume of care and the hospital's deficit are computed, as percentages of the total volume of care and total ambulatory care service deficits for all participating hospitals. These are then put together in a weighted formula which gives more importance to size of patient load and degree of contract compliance than it does to the size of the deficit, and the proportion of the total amount of money available for that contract year which goes to the particular hospital is arrived at.

This system is rather complicated, and there is a danger that it could become very rigid and bureaucratic. However, it is also a very creative new departure which attempts to relate payments directly and objectively to performance. As such, it really deserves a fair trial with rigorous, objective evaluation.

Unfortunately, in October 1975, the waters were muddied when, in the midst of its financial crisis, the city stopped its monetary contributions to the ACP. This complicated the questions of inspection, contract enforcement, and method of dividing up the available funds, of course. The program was able to continue financially, through Section 39.3 (2) of the State Health Code (see App. 8), which provides for dollar-for-dollar state matching of philanthropic contributions made to individual institutions for the purpose of operating programs covered by Sections 39 and 40 of the code. Interestingly enough, even though it no longer provided funds, the city still carried out the inspections, and controlled the flow of state money. Let us say that after making its inspection and applying the compliance formula, the city determines that the hospital is entitled to a $400,000 subsidy, $200,000 of which would be state money. The hospital can receive the $200,000 if it matches the amount with philanthropic contributions. However, even if the hospital can raise more than that amount in contributions, it can receive no more state money than it would be entitled to, using the compliance formula, if the city were still putting up its share. In sum, the total amount of money in the pot is double the state appropriation for the year. Each participating hospital's potential share is determined by inspection, and application of the compliance formula. The hospital can get the state money to which it is entitled by dollar-for-dollar matching with philanthropic contributions.

As would be expected, there were strong demands from the voluntary hospitals to remove the city from the inspection process and deal directly with the state (Pomrinse, 1976). Of course, the State Health Department has never been involved with the ACP inspection program, and has not shown much interest in it. As of the summer of 1976, the situation had not changed, and the City Health Department was maintaining its role in the inspection process and the determination of the distribution of funds. In the spring of 1977, however, the ACP appeared to have come to an end. The State disbanded the City Health Department's inspection unit, and the Governor proposed a budget with no Ghetto Medicine money in it.

References

Bellin, L. E. Interview, New York, N.Y., Mar. 12, 1975.
Bellin, L. E., et al. Phase one of consumer participation in policies of 22 voluntary hospitals in New York City. *American Journal of Public Health*, 1972, *62*, 1370.
Bernstein, G. Interview, North Woodmere, N.Y., Mar. 10, 1975.
Borsody, R. Interview, New York, N.Y., July 12, 1976.

Consumer Commission on the Accreditation of Health Services. Ambulatory care program: A role for the consumer. *Health Perspectives*, January/February 1975, 2, (1).

Fearon, Z. Interviews, New York, N.Y., Apr. 4, 1975, July 12, 1976.

Gambuti, G. Interview, New York, N.Y., Mar. 25, 1975.

Hammerling, A. Interview, New York, N.Y., Apr. 2, 1975.

McCann, M. F. *The ambulatory care program: A manual for consumers.* New York: Community Health Institute, 1974.

Metsch, J. M. Unpublished doctoral dissertation, University of North Carolina, August 1972.

Metsch, J. M., & Veney, J. E. A model of adaptive behavior of hospital administrators to the mandate to implement consumer participation. *Medical Care*, 1974, *12*, 338.

New York City Health Department. *Guidelines for implementation of Chapter 967, Laws of 1968: Schedule* A. New York, N.Y. June 1974. Process.

New York City Health Department, Bureau of Ambulatory Care. *Explanation of formula for determination of subsidy, Commissioner's monthly meeting.* May 1975. Process.

New York City Health Department, Medical Assistance Program, Division of Institutional Ambulatory and Acute Care Services. *Compliance determination: Summary and index* (Document No. VH–18). New York: 1975–76.

Pomrinse, S. D. Interview, New York, N.Y., April 4, 1975.

Pomrinse, S. D. *Statement.* Paper presented at public hearing, Assembly Standing Committee on Health, Program Subcommittee on Community-Based and Ambulatory Care, New York, February 12, 1976.

Reichman, S. Interview, New York, N.Y., Apr. 4, 1975.

Schwarz, A. Interviews, New York, N.Y., Mar. 12 and Apr. 16, 1975, July 12, 1976, and subsequent telephone conversations.

Schwarz, A., & Furman, R. *Evaluation process in ambulatory care: The Ghetto Medicine Program.* New York City Health Department, February 1975. Process.

Schwarz, A., et al. A Ghetto Medicine program. *Social Work*, November 1973, p. 90.

Schwarz, A., et al. *Evaluating ambulatory care in New York City.* New York City Department of Health, June 1973. Process.

Travers, T. Interview, New York, N.Y., July 12, 1976.

United Hospital Fund of New York. *Workbook for the study of ambulatory care in New York City.* New York: no date (presumably 1975).

Wainfeld, B. Interview, Brooklyn, N.Y., March 26, 1975.

7

Ghetto Medicine in Suffolk County

Introduction

A few of the counties in the state of New York have attempted to develop programs along the lines of the original Ghetto Medicine concepts: Albany, Erie, Monroe, Westchester, Nassau, and Suffolk. According to Andrew Fleck (1975), the program did not generally catch on because of three factors: (1) The 1968–69 Medicaid cutbacks sharply reduced the available third-party reimbursement for local health department general medical services, thus increasing the amounts which local governments would have had to supply from their general revenues, even though matched by the State. (2) Local health departments do not comprise "accounting entities" within their jurisdictions. Thus incoming funds disappear into general revenues, and it is difficult to establish an identifiable program. (3) Local health officers were not very interested.

In 1975, there were five County Health Department health centers in Suffolk County. Three of them, the South Brookhaven Health Center in Mastic Beach, the Martin Luther King Health Center in Wyandanch, and the Brentwood Family Health Center in Brentwood, are operated by local hospitals under contract funded through the Ghetto Medicine program. They were all in or near poverty areas. In this report, two of them are discussed. The South Brook-

This chapter is based principally upon the work of Virginia Neary. The material was gathered primarily from interviews in the spring of 1975 with Mary McLaughin, M.D., Leo Gitman, M.D., Oliver Schepers, Bessie Uhrquart, and Paul O'Brien of the Suffolk County Department of Health Services; visits to the Mastic Beach and Wyandanch Health Centers with staff interviews there, and discussions with community representatives on the community advisory boards to the Martin Luther King and Mastic Beach Health Centers.

haven Health Center is the most easterly and is in the most rural community of the three centers. The residents of the surrounding area are predominantly white, and there is a relatively large proportion of elderly people. The center's services are provided through family practice clinics by general practitioners and specialists in family medicine. The Martin Luther King Center is the most westerly one. The surrounding area is relatively heavily populated. The residents of Wyandanch are predominantly black, and there is a high proportion of low-income families. The services at the Martin Luther King Center are organized around specialty clinics. Primary care is provided through pediatric and adult medicine clinics by pediatricians and internists.

HISTORY AND BACKGROUND OF HEALTH CENTERS
IN SUFFOLK COUNTY

At the beginning of the sixties, the Suffolk County government provided almost no organized ambulatory care services. Chest clinics and orthopedic diagnostic clinics were the only personal public health services available. The Health Department was not interested in expanding ambulatory services, and private physicians opposed county involvement in general health care services. However, public health nurses working in the county were aware of the fact that many families lacked access to private physicians because of geographical distance and/or the inability to pay. Most of the medical attention received by such families was episodic and obtained at hospital emergency rooms. Even well-baby care was not available, and there were many children in low-income areas who were not immunized.

In 1964, the first well-baby clinics were established. There were four of them, in Huntington, Farmingville, Bay Shore, and Riverhead. Most of the organizing, scheduling, and actual patient care was done by public health nurses, who were the prime movers behind the establishment of the clinics. Several others were established later. Well-baby clinics, however, were only authorized to provide preventive care. When parents brought in sick children, they had to be told that the clinic could not treat them and that they should see their private physician. Since many of the families were attending the well-baby clinic precisely because they had no family physician, this advice seemed almost absurd. Often sick children went without care, or they were seen at hospital emergency rooms. When private physicians were sought for sick patients from the well-baby clinics, there was often negative feedback to the clinics such as "If you can take them when they're well, you can take them when they're sick."

In 1966, the Office of the Suffolk Executive became increasingly concerned with the problems of health care for the residents of Suffolk County. The office commissioned a study of the feasibility of establishing a county hospital. The study concluded that the county was too big and the population too dispersed to make a county hospital either economically viable or of much use to the population. One of the recommendations was that, as an alternative, the county should support the establishment of a series of ambulatory care centers. Areas of particular need were designated.

The first health center established in Suffolk County designed to provide a full range of treatment services was the Martin Luther King Center in Wyandanch, opened in July 1968. Planning that had been underway for such a center was speeded up in response to rioting in the community. Furthermore, the Ghetto Medicine program had just been created, and the plan for the center was designed to take advantage of it.

Over a period of time, the County Executive's Office began to realize, partially through community pressure, that there was a need for health centers in other communities. The Brentwood Family Health Center, also established under Ghetto Medicine, developed in a patchwork fashion. First came a well-baby clinic at Southside Hospital in Bay Shore, a neighboring community to Brentwood. A pediatric treatment clinic was opened in Brentwood proper in 1970, and in the same year, a prenatal clinic was started at Southside. Finally, in 1971 the county contracted with Southside Hospital to provide and expand services at the Brentwood location. All the services formerly at Southside were moved to Brentwood, and the Family Health Center was born.

The South Brookhaven Health Center in Mastic Beach was established in response to community pressure. A health council formed by South Brookhaven (township) area residents in the late 1960s was sophisticated in its knowledge of the needs of the area and was able to articulate them well. The greatest concentration of need was actually in the village of Patchogue, more densely populated and having a higher percentage of low-income residents than Mastic Beach. However, the closing by the State Health Department in 1972 of the Bayview Hospital, a small twenty-nine bed proprietary hospital in Mastic Beach, provided a ready-made facility for the health center. The community health council was opposed to the location because it was out of the way but eventually compromised since the selection of an alternative site would have delayed the opening of the center. A second health facility, the South Brookhaven Health Center West, opened in Patchogue in late 1975.

In addition to the three Ghetto Medicine centers, the county operates health centers in Amityville and Riverhead, which also provide general medical services, primarily to low-income patients. They are funded through different mechanisms.

Administration

The Suffolk County Health Services Department is responsible for overall operations of the health center program. Direction and responsibility is split between the Office of the Assistant Commissioner for Administration, the Office of Program Evaluation and Research, and the Division of Patient Care. For most services, the department operates its Ghetto Medicine health centers by the contract method. The Good Samaritan Hospital operates the King Center, the Southside Hospital, Brentwood, and the Brookhaven Memorial Hospital, South Brookhaven. Hospitals are reimbursed for all direct costs of operation plus 10 percent for administration. Certain services, however, such as public health nursing, family planning, and social work are provided directly by the county. Some community outreach services are provided by contract between the Health Services Department and the County Economic Opportunity Commission. Thus, at any one center there can be employees of several different agencies or institutions.

The contract between the county and the hospitals is quite similar to the first New York City Ghetto Medicine contracts. A variety of program and staffing requirements are described. Operating standards for the clinics are given in quite a bit of detail in "Exhibit A," while the guidelines for the Community Advisory Boards are contained in "Exhibit B." These are similar in concept to the schedules of the present New York City contract, but, in general, the Suffolk contract has about the same degree of precision and detail as the early New York City contract (see Appendix 12).

The New York State Department of Health has generally maintained the same distant relationship to both the administration and evaluation of Suffolk County's Ghetto Medicine program that it has in relation to New York City's ACP.

FINANCING

The total costs of the health centers under the Ghetto Medicine program since its inception in 1968 through 1974 were $5,351,883 (Table 7–1). Data on patient revenues are available only for 1973 and 1974, when they were $380,986 and $535,222 respectively, about 25 percent of total cost each year. The major revenue sources are Medicaid and Medicare. New York State reimburses the county for quite a bit less than 50 percent of operating deficits since in fiscal 1975, the sole year for which figures were available, the state spent only approximately $250,000 in Suffolk County for Ghetto Medicine.

TABLE 7–1

Cost of Health Center Operations,
Suffolk County Ghetto Medicine Program, 1968–74

| YEAR | HOSPITAL | | | |
	Martin Luther King	*South Brookhaven*	*Brentwood*	*Total*
1968	$ 98,321	$ —	$ —	$ 98,321
1969	206,786	—	—	206,786
1970	246,739	—	—	246,739
1971	335,377	—	61,186	396,563
1972	422,072	49,588	209,258	680,918
1973	536,529	528,799	616,203	1,681,531
1974	545,725	565,900	929,400	2,041,025
Total	$2,391,548	$1,144,288	$1,816,047	$5,351,883

SOURCE: Suffolk County Department of Health Services, Hauppauge, N.Y., 1975.

EVALUATION PROCEDURES

In 1975, Suffolk County was early on in the development of its evaluation procedures. It had no formal mechanism for enforcement of the health center contract and apparently little had been done to date to develop one. The Suffolk County facility evaluation protocol followed the structural approach and was concerned with the following: (1) Governing bodies and management; (2) Administrative structure and planning; (3) Staffing patterns; (4) Community Advisory Board; (5) Physical plant and environment; (6) Service profile; (7) Medical records; (8) Statistics. There was no medical auditing program. The department was working on the development of a system of medical audit based on Kessner's tracer method. Both the facility evaluation protocol and the tracer system were still in the preliminary stages of development. However, the system planned thus far does not contemplate community involvement in evaluation.

COMMUNITY ADVISORY COMMITTEES

All the health centers under the Ghetto Medicine program have Community Advisory Committees in order to provide community input into health center policies and operations, and to ensure that the health center administration and staff is responsive to the needs of the community. The role and the political stance of the committees vary from center to center depending on both the composition of the committee and on the hospital involved. The County Health Department's Division of Patient Care has developed guidelines for the Community Advisory Committees to delineate what the division thinks the community role in health center operations should be.

The Community Advisory Committees do not appear to have anything like the contract-enforcing powers of the New York City Community Boards.

Health Center Operations

THE MARTIN LUTHER KING HEALTH CENTER

The Martin Luther King Health Center is located in Wyandanch, a predominantly black community with a high percentage of low-income residents. In 1968, the area had a large deficit in health, recreational, and other facilities. It is still a depressed area. The building occupied by the center is in a shopping plaza, occupies 4,300 square feet, and is severely overcrowded. The State Health Department has cited the building for safety hazards. There is no conference room and virtually no administrative office space. A request for the addition of a 1,200-square-foot mobile unit has been approved by the county, but as of June 1975 the unit existed only on paper.

Management is rather complex. There is no full-time administrator. Walter J. O'Connor, M.D., from the staff of the contractee, Good Samaritan Hospital, is Medical Director responsible for overall administration, and he also serves in his clinical capacity as a pediatrician. However, there are several different employers for health center personnel, including the county. Various employees have different rates of pay, different vacation and holiday schedules, and are responsible to different organizations. Coordination and the development of an integrated program is difficult under such conditions.

Anyone who resides in Suffolk County can be a patient at any health center. Although there is a defined geographic catchment area, no patients are turned away because they reside outside the area. In 1974, the county did implement a system to obtain accurate information as to where the majority of health center patients reside. It is O'Connor's feeling that the majority of patients come from the Wyandanch area, with the exception of obstetric and gynecological patients. Martin Luther King is the only health center which offers obstetrics and gynecology, and women come from great distance to attend that clinic.

The total number of patient visits to the health center in 1974 was 22,499 (Table 7–2). Utilization has more than doubled since the center first opened, but it is still not a very large operation. Growth has halted, due primarily to lack of space. The center already operates from 9 A.M. to 9 P.M. Mondays through Thursdays and 9 A.M. to 5 P.M. on Fridays.

TABLE 7–2

Utilization of Services, King Health Center,
Suffolk County, N.Y., 1968–74

SERVICE	1968	1969	1970	1971	1972	1973	1974
General							
pediatrics	3,686	7,511	7,784	9,064	8,399	8,111	7,968
Head Start							
Outreach	—	—	—	—	28[a]	71	—
Allergy	—	406	1,227	959	2,628	3,419	2,846
ENT	—	—	—	—	—	65	93
Cardiac	18	80	66	92	44	80	88
Adult							
medicine	—	774	2,144	4,914	5,869	5,923	5,847
OBS/GYN	194	1,306	1,875	1,915	2,419	2,203	2,333
Pap smear	—	—	—	185	1,106	823	238
Sickle cell test							
& counseling	—	—	—	—	49	61	73
Subtotal GSH-							
staffed clinics	3,898	10,007	13,096	17,129	20,542	20,756	19,955
Alcohol clinic	—	—	376	333	463	346	n.a.
Family planning	157	656	828	1,463	1,704	2,088	2,544
Mental health	—	44	462	190	—	—	—
Total visits	4,055	10,777	14,762	19,115	22,709	23,190	22,499

SOURCE: Suffolk County Department of Health Services, Hauppauge, N.Y., 1975.
[a]Included in general pediatrics before December 1973.

There is no transportation provided for patients to get to the health center. It is the county's goal eventually to have a transportation component at all the health centers, but so far it has not been implemented at all of them. Medicaid patients who are certified as in need of transportation can be reimbursed for their travel expenses. There is little public transportation in Suffolk, and undoubtedly this factor keeps some people from obtaining medical care.

General adult medical and pediatric services are offered during most clinic sessions. There are also several sessions for obstetrics-gynecology and family planning, and allergy. Preventive medicine programs in the form of venereal disease screening, pap smears, sickle-cell testing and the like are offered under the auspices of different agencies. In 1974, the county introduced a limited amount of dental service into the health center program in the form of a dental van which rotates among the centers.

For specialty services not available at Martin Luther King, an informal arrangement was made with certain specialists on the staff of Good Samaritan Hospital. However, no arrangements were made with regard to fees. The doctors accept Medicaid patients. However, there are a large number of health center families not eligible for Medicaid but too poor to pay a specialist's fee. As far as could be ascertained, no provisions had been made to deal with this situation.

The physicians on the staff of Martin Luther King are all board-certified specialists. There are about four full-time equivalent physicians, internists and pediatricians. The health center program constantly faces problems obtaining qualified physicians. The goal is to completely eliminate sessional physicians in favor of salaried personnel. However, county salaries are not high, and recruiting is difficult.

The nursing staff consists of a nurse coordinator (who is a pediatric nurse practitioner), a head nurse, an obstetric nurse practitioner, a registered nurse, two licensed practical nurses, and several aides. In addition, the Health Department's Public Health Nursing Staff works directly with the Health Center staff in many areas. Health center nurses play a vital role in many aspects of total patient care and provide a great deal of direct service. The King Center was working on the development of a system of provider teams. It uses nurse practitioners. Before 1975, much of the nurses' time was consumed with answering phones, scheduling appointments, and arranging referrals. However, the hiring of a unit clerk in nursing freed the nursing staff from clerical duties and allowed them to become more actively involved in patient care.

Routine laboratory tests are done on site at the health center. More elaborate tests are done at the hospital or outside laboratories. Radiology services are available at the health center five days per week, including two evening sessions. Good Samaritan Hospital provides back-up for procedures which the center cannot perform. The shortage of space in the medical records room was perhaps more acute than in any other area of the center. If not more acute, it was at least more obvious. There was virtually no space for new records. A medical records clerk joked about suspending racks from the ceiling in order to accommodate the overflow.

The Social Services Department of the King Center is administered directly by the county. The Social Services Department is involved in the following areas of practice: (1) Direct service to patients; (2) Information and referral; (3) Counseling—Individual and family; (4) Crisis intervention; (5) Interagency communication and community organization.

THE VIEW OF THE COMMUNITY ADVISORY BOARD

At a meeting of the King Center's Community Advisory Board, the issue which surfaced repeatedly was the perceived failure of the county to follow through on its obligations and commitments. The long promised mobile unit designed to temporarily alleviate the space problems at the center had still not arrived in the spring of 1975. O'Connor informed the committee that the latest delay was due to the fact that Babylon Town, in which the community of Wyandanch is located, has an ordinance prohibiting trailers. The county promised to attempt to obtain clearance from the town for the Health Center mobile unit, but so far had done nothing. The Advisory Committee was furious at the new delay, and the issue of the county bureaucracy and problems in dealing with it was discussed at length.

The Advisory Committee expressed complete satisfaction with the hospital. The general feeling was that the hospital was trying its best to provide good quality health services, in the face of innumerable county obstacles. The biggest problem is lack of space and the overcrowding that results. This again was traced back to the county and its failure for three years to find and authorize a new building for the center. Lack of equipment and supplies, also attributed to the county, was another problem mentioned.

The Advisory Committee has been involved to a limited extent in personnel decisions at the center. There is a Grievance Committee which is responsible for bringing patients' complaints to the attention of the full committee and the center administration. At this particular meeting, none were reported.

O'Connor was very active in the committee meeting, especially in discussing problems with the County Health Department. He explained that the only way the center has been able to get needed personnel, equipment, repairs, etc., has been to threaten to close down. He employed this tactic twice in the first four months of 1974, and both times it worked.

The Community Advisory Committee and the Health Center administration appear to work closely together. The committee voiced its complete satisfaction with the hospital, and seems to view it as an ally against the county bureaucracy. It is impossible to say whether this is an independent judgment, or whether it is the result of control of the Advisory Committee by the Health Center administration.

Summary. In summary, the King Center is small, active, overcrowded, confusingly administered, and trying hard, with more hindrance than help from the county. Except for the fact that the center is operated in the main under contract rather than directly by the county, serving as it does an area greatly underserved in the past, it is in fact doing what the original framers of the Ghetto Medicine program had in mind. However, the contract enforcement program is nothing like that in New York City, so one has little to go on in assessing the quality of the product.

SOUTH BROOKHAVEN HEALTH CENTER

The South Brookhaven Health Center is located in the building that formerly housed the Bayview Hospital in Mastic Beach, New York, notably out of the way and difficult to find. The center opened on October 9, 1972. The health center building is large and spacious, especially when compared with the King Center. However, hospital rooms and layout are not well suited to health center operations. Suffolk County moved very slowly on necessary renovations, and in 1975 they were still far from completed. There were also severe delays in the provision of needed office and medical equipment and supplies. The parking lot and access roads were in very poor condition.

The center, administered by the Department of Community Medicine at the Brookhaven Memorial Hospital in Patchogue, has a full-time Medical Director and Administrator. There is a Nurse Coordinator, responsible to the Administrator, who supervises the nursing staff. Nevertheless, the South Brookhaven Center has the same complex administrative organization as does the King Center, due to the fact that services are provided by multiple agencies. Outreach is provided by the county's Economic Opportunity Commission (EOC). There is a county-operated family planning service which is also provided by the EOC. The County Dental Van provides limited dental services. The local District Public Health Nursing Station is located in the center. Mental health services are provided by the Central Islip State Hospital Aftercare Clinic which is housed in the center. The Social Worker is hired and paid by the county. There is a transportation service, provided directly by the County Department of Transportation. Again, an administrative quagmire.

In the spring of 1975, there was a twelve-to-fourteen-week wait for an appointment for physical examination. For other appointments there was a ten-week wait. Due to the long wait for appointments, there was a large volume of walk-in patients, and a screening nurse was hired to do triage, with some patients sent to the Emergency Room of the Brookhaven Memorial Hospital.

There was a total of 27,552 patient visits at the center in 1974. This is more than double the 11,437 which had been provided as of September 1973, after one full year of operation. The opening of the second site at Patchogue was not expected to reduce utilization, since only approximately 15 percent of the center's patients were from within the Patchogue catchment area. Ninety percent of the patients are white, reflecting the racial composition of the area, 62 percent self-pay on a sliding-fee scale, with the balance about equally divided between Medicaid and Medicare. Sixty-five percent of the patients live in the immediate vicinity.

Medical service is provided by family physicians, an internist, and a pediatrician in Family Practice clinics. There are no specialty clinics at the center. Dental work-up, vision screening, and family planning are done as part of family practice. The only services that are provided categorically at South Brookhaven are those not delivered under the contract with the Brookhaven Memorial Hospital, which are provided by other agencies.

The Health Center has an active Community Advisory Committee which is involved in major health center decisions, including the hiring and firing of supervisory personnel, including the Administrator, the Medical Director, and the Nurse Coordinator. All other personnel decisions are left to the Administrator. From the committee's point of view, the biggest problems in providing quality services at the health center were delays in obtaining from the county promised new personnel, equipment, supplies, renovations, and repairs, due, they felt, to county "red tape and bureaucracy," as at the King Center.

The Advisory Committee felt that it has a good working relationship with the hospital, though there have been times of disagreement when the committee felt that it had to stand firm for its interests. The committee generally felt that good quality services were being provided and that the supervision by the hospital was good, although, as might be assumed from the lengthy delays in obtaining new appointments, they were not entirely satisfied with the quantity of service. Overall, the committee felt that the center was making progress toward the goal of providing comprehensive health care, although it was still a long way from achieving that goal. Just as at the King Center, the Board felt the County obstruction was the chief obstacle to be overcome.

Future Directions

In broad terms, the county intends "to continue the development of ambulatory health centers until quality primary medical care is available to all segments of the population and to develop the comprehensiveness of these centers according to the guidelines established by the New York State Public Health Laws." A minimum of four new centers were being planned for completion in the seventies. The Health Services Department wants to increase the availability of transportation so that all the centers will be able to provide transportation to and from the center for patients who are in need. Expansion of the hours of coverage is another priority. By the end of the seventies, it is hoped that all of the centers will be open twelve hours daily, six days per week. In addition, telephone consultation will be available when the centers are closed. It is the aim of the Health Services Department to reduce to a minimum the use of hospital emergency rooms for nonemergent problems by health center patients.

A Health Center Coordinating Council was formed in 1972 to pursue the prospects of regional planning among the health centers. Eventually it is planned that each center will have all necessary specialty services. However, that time is still well in the future. In the meantime, regionalization of specialty services will avoid unnecessary duplication of some and absence of others. Telephone answering services and personnel coverage during hours when the health centers are closed could also be effectively pooled. So far, the centers have been grouped into regions, but little else has been accomplished along these lines.

We have now seen in some detail what a program operated by a county under one variation, the contract mechanism, of the provisions of the original Ghetto Medicine program looks like. Interesting it is. Like Biggs's conception of 1920, it isn't.

8

Ghetto Medicine:
Discussions of the Findings

The State Health Department
and Ghetto Medicine

The New York State Health Department created the Ghetto Medicine program. In effect it brought to life part of the conception
which Herman Biggs had developed forty-five years earlier, although
it was not nearly as grand as the Biggs design, which had included
inpatient and integrated preventive services as well as ambulatory
general medical services, in health department centers. However,
the program did not come off as planned, and the department seemed
to lose interest. Only six counties outside of New York City chose
to participate in the program. A statewide string of nonhospital general medical clinics in underserved areas, which could have been
like contemporary neighborhood health centers but under local government rather than community or hospital sponsorship, did not
spring up. There are no State Health Department summaries of
Ghetto Medicine activities. In four Annual Reports, which are admittedly skimpy, for 1969 and 1971–73, there is no mention of Ghetto
Medicine. There is no evidence that the department has ever attempted to enforce the Ghetto Medicine regulations in the Health
Code, except for the state aid formula. There are no publications
by State Health Department officials on Ghetto Medicine.

As with Article 28, the state legislature has also had little interest. The first time the Assembly Health Committee considered activities of either the state or any local health department under
Ghetto Medicine was on February 12, 1976, when one day of hearings were held by its Program Sub-Committee on Community-Based
and Ambulatory Care. The Joint Legislative Committee on Public

Health, etc. (see chap. 4) did hold one set of hearings on Ghetto Medicine on October 24–25, 1968. However, transcripts of those hearings were not published, although transcripts of other hearings held over the years by the committee were readily available. In its 1969 Annual Report, the Joint Committee devoted nine brief paragraphs to Ghetto Medicine, consisting primarily of a legislative history.

Ghetto Medicine has thus become primarily a New York City program, the Ambulatory Care Program. One of the most striking features of the ACP is the degree to which the State Health Department ignores it, aside from paying its share of the cost. This seems to have held true even when the city is no longer putting up any money. One of our most significant and most disturbing findings concerns the chasm which exists between the Health Departments of New York State and New York City. The enmity is notable. To listen to representatives of each department and their respective partisans outside of government talk, virtually all of the leadership in the other agency are: (1) dumb; (2) ignorant; (3) the cause of all the troubles of the interviewee's own agency. "If only those people would . . . ," the refrain goes on both sides: (1) "shut up and listen"; (2) "understand *our* problems"; (3) "inform themselves of what is going on"; (4) "learn the meaning of a dollar"; and so on.

This is highly unfortunate. Both departments have great powers and responsibilities. Both departments have great pioneering histories, interestingly enough, having had Herman Biggs as a former Commissioner. If the departments could somehow be brought to work together, a great deal more could be accomplished for the health of the people of the whole state of New York. Unfortunately, the barriers to such a development are high, and we know only part of the story. Party politics would appear to be very important in maintaining the split. Both departments have strong civil service traditions, but the top leadership in both are always political appointees. The Governor of New York State is more often that not a Republican while the Mayor of New York City is more often than not a Democrat or, in the case of John Lindsay, a maverick Republican who certainly did not get along at all with the incumbent Governor. However, relationships do not seem to have improved much since 1974, when both the Governor's mansion and City Hall were occupied by Democrats. Then there is the age-old struggle over the question of home rule for New York City. Under the Constitution, besides the federal government only the states have inherent sovereignty. Any sovereignty which cities have is given to them by state legislatures and can be easily taken away. In health, what powers the City Health Department has are given to it by the State Health Department and can be taken away with ease. Such a situation does not make for good feelings, nor does it encourage cooperation. Nevertheless, whatever the history, the outcome is unfortunate.

The Ambulatory Care Program in New York City

PROGRAM ACHIEVEMENTS

We found the ACP a fascinating program. It is creative. It is apparently productive. It achieved certain changes in the operations of voluntary hospital clinics in New York City for relatively small outlays of funds. In fact, one of the most amazing things about it is the extent to which hospitals will go in changing, attempting to change, or at least appearing to change, in order to get an amount of money which is relatively small in proportion to their total budgets. It makes one wonder what they would do if they had to make changes to get large amounts of money.

In objective terms, New York City has been somewhat better, but not too much better, in carrying out evaluations of the ACP than the state has been in carrying out evaluations of the Article 28 program. Clear goals for the program were stated in the first prototype contract, and there have been periodic although episodic attempts by the Bureau of Ambulatory Care to measure achievement of these goals. There is still no ongoing objective evaluation program. Although the academic literature concerning the ACP is not voluminous, at least there *is* one, descriptive and evaluative, produced by persons both inside and outside the City Department of Health. The City Department is concerned with the problem of establishing that there are connections between the ACP and improvements in the health care of the people of New York City. One does not get that feeling at the state level in reference to Article 28.

The major point in consideration of the effects of the ACP, however, is this. Despite the lack of operational, clear, objective evaluation mechanisms, which are certainly needed, the subjective view of almost everyone interviewed is that the program is working and producing positive results. In our view, when hospital directors, hospital ambulatory care directors, Health Department officials, and community representatives all agree that the program is a success and is producing positive results, indeed it must be doing something right. In contrast, in discussions around Article 28 implementation, one does not get anything like that feeling at all.

QUALITY CONTROL IN HOSPITAL AMBULATORY CARE

The ACP has challenged the basis of the whole structure of the participating voluntary hospitals in New York City in two vitally important areas: quality control and ambulatory care. Hospitals have been forced to look at two of their prize stepchildren and make some changes. For quite some time, under two general approaches to quality control, accreditation and licensing, hospitals have accepted outside agency audits of the quality of the care provided on the basis of structural standards. However, hospitals—or, more specifically, their medical staffs—have traditionally maintained the position that quality auditing using specific approaches which examine discrete instances of health care delivery was the private province of the medical staff alone and that anything else would be "interference with the practice of medicine." The ACP, which uses process as well as structural standards in its auditing procedures, and thus looks at discrete instances of care delivery, has cracked this barrier and has probably cracked it once and for all.

CHANGES IN HOSPITAL MODE OF OPERATIONS

One of the most significant features of the ACP is that it has introduced the principle of the contract mechanism to control the transfer of government money to private institutions to support their own services. Private institutions have contracted with government before of course, but it always has been for money to run a program *someplace else,* an affiliated municipal hospital, a neighborhood health center, a drug program, or the like. ACP money is for the hospital's own operations. Of course, the major amounts of government monies coming into hospitals, under the Medicare and Medicaid programs, come in on a cost-reimbursement, item-of-service basis. The contrast is striking.

Further, the ACP has introduced meaningful community participation into hospital operations. Many of us who struggled through the "community control" issue in reference to neighborhood health centers and municipal hospitals came away with a rather jaundiced view of the whole affair (Jonas, 1971). The ACP presents a mode of what can be called meaningful community participation. The conflict over "who is in charge here," which afflicted many a neighborhood health center for many years, is clearly dealt with. The contracting hospital is in charge of the operation program. The City Health Department is in charge of the money and the inspections. The Community Board is in charge of contract enforcement, relating both to contractor and contractee. This is different, creative, productive of positive change, and has potential for wide application.

The ACP requires maintenance of effort on the part of the participating hospitals in return for receiving money, thus mandating minimum volumes of care. There was a significant lowering of financial barriers to care for the "near-poor." There is the requirement for publication of ACP inspection reports. In contrast, it is only recently that Article 28 inspection reports have come into the public domain. In further contrast, on May 30, 1975, the JCAH filed a suit against the Secretary of the United States Department of Health, Education, and Welfare to bar him from releasing JCAH accreditation reports to the public (*Hospital Week*, 1975). The ACP requires not only program audits but also fiscal accounting, with those reports being made public as well. Finally, the compliance formula directly links level and quality of performance to payment. These steps are all significant changes in general hospital operations resulting from the ACP.

CHANGES IN HOSPITAL AMBULATORY CARE
RESULTING FROM THE ACP

First, the ACP kept the voluntary hospital clinics open. If one takes the hospitals at their word, without the ACP many of them would have been forced to close their clinics for financial reasons. In terms of more basic change, hospitals are being forced to reorient their basic thinking on the organization, structure, and place in the hospital hierarchy of ambulatory services. These changes are not taking place overnight, but they are taking place and, in long-range historical terms, they are significant. In dealing with the place of ambulatory care in hospitals, it must be recalled that very strong historical traditions are being dealt with. One is the charitable institution tradition of "taking care of the poor," always much stronger on the outpatient than on the inpatient side, particularly in the last forty years with the growth of hospitalization insurance. A second is the basis of attending medical staff participation in the clinics as part of their "obligation" to the hospital. A third is the stress given to teaching and research in traditional teaching hospital ambulatory services at the expense of patient service. A fourth is the traditional tripartite, vertical organizational structure of hospital ambulatory services, which militates against planning and implementing comprehensive services. The ACP deals with these four powerful historical trends and is making strides in changing them.

Most observers felt also that specific improvements have been made in hospital ambulatory services. Among them, not necessarily in order of importance, are: the requirement for a Director of Ambulatory Care; the institution of an appointment system; the removal of interns from emergency rooms; the requirement for primary care physicians and the implementation of the concept of comprehensive care; reduction in the number of specialty clinics; increased social services; the introduction of patient drug profiles; the institution of nurse conferencing.

Problems do remain in areas which have been the toughest nuts to crack in hospital ambulatory services: the limited authority of the directors of ambulatory care; the medical records system, with lost charts and unposted test results; lengthy, although reduced, patient waiting times; long delays in first appointments for new patients.

THE INSPECTION PROCESS

A number of interviewees pointed out problems in the inspection process. The inspections are done with relative frequency, but they are done relatively quickly, one day at a time. There does seem to be a shortage of staff. Hospitals are idiosyncratic, and so are ambulatory services. There are complaints from the hospitals of lack of direct operational experience and lack of knowledge of "what it's really like" on the part of inspectors. It is our feeling that some distance between inspectors and inspectees is necessary if objectivity is to be maintained, but difficulties arising from the lack of appreciation of nuance are real, too.

One possible way of dealing with this problem would be to introduce an element of peer review into the inspection process, requiring that one or two members of each inspection team be drawn from the staffs of participating hospitals, on a rotating basis. The JCAH experience has clearly indicated the problems of quality review systems entirely dependent on peer review. However, the mixed approach could be productive. Another approach which might be considered would be to require hospitals to do a complete self-evaluation, using the official protocols, before the regular inspection is undertaken. The comparison of self-rating with outside rating on the central question of contract compliance could be most enlightening to all concerned.

LEGAL STANDING OF THE ACP

One of the most amazing things about the ACP, particularly in contrast with the picture of Article 28 implementation, is how much has been done in a program with such questionable legal standing. The ACP cannot be said to hang by a thread. The support is more like a gossamer strand, almost critics might refer to it as a spider's web for catching unwary hospitals. The ACP was created from the original Ghetto Medicine program by Governor Rockefeller to bail out financially ailing voluntary hospitals, with no clear basis in law for doing so, although the contracting mechanism, for *health centers*, was in the regulations. The ACP has never been embodied in state law, nor in state regulations. Nor has it ever appeared in city law or health code. It is maintained from year to year by contracts and state/city appropriations. We must say it again: Amazing!

QUALITY CONTROL UNDER THE ACP AND MEDICAID

It is interesting to compare the approach to quality control undertaken by the City Health Department under the ACP with the approach which they used to carry out their quality control responsibilities under the New York State Medicaid program.[1] In 1968, Lowell Bellin, who at that time was Executive Medical Director for the City Health Department's Medicaid program, said:

> What is exhilaratingly revolutionary about Medicaid is neither the program's more generous enrollment of the medically indigent, nor even its delightful smorgasbord of comprehensive health services. No, Medicaid's critical innovation lurks elsewhere—in its exclusive assignment to the Health Department of the heady tasks of standard setting, surveillance, and enforcement of quality in every aspect and every locus of publicly funded personal health care. (1969, p. 820)

This was a statement of high principle, and it was accompanied by others (Alexander, 1969; Bellin and Kavaler, 1969; Kavaler, 1969; O'Rourke, 1969). It appeared as if, for the first time, there would be a wide-ranging medical care quality control program, applied to all providers, and implicitly, using a variety of auditing techniques.

What in fact happened has been somewhat different. Over the years, the department has concentrated its efforts on catching the out-and-out cheaters, the gross overutilizers, among the providers, often in an effort to save or recover money (*New York Times*, August 4, 1971; January 9, 1972; April 19, 1975). The Medicaid quality-control program has taken on many aspects of a "policing" effort, and indeed that is the first word in the title of the 1969 Bellin-Kavaler paper (1969). Thus the program has concentrated its efforts on finding the relatively small proportion of providers who do cheat: overbill, bill for nonexistent services, prescribe unnecessary treatment, and the like.

Potentially far more serious, in our view, are the problems in the quality of medical care given to the vast majority of Medicaid patients by the vast majority of Medicaid providers who don't cheat. This area has not received much attention. It is not known whether the bulk of care given by individual providers and paid for by

1. This text was written long before the New York City Medicaid scandals of the fall of 1976 ("Senator Moss . . . Sees Medicaid Abuse in New York City," *New York Times*, Aug. 30, 1976). It is not predicated on any material revealed by them, although that material certainly supports the conclusions herein stated.

Medicaid is good, bad, or indifferent. Nor, in striking contrast to the ACP, has the quality of care provided in institutions receiving Medicaid money had much if any attention. An institution receiving a few hundred thousand dollars under the ACP is inspected regularly and thoroughly by the Bureau of Ambulatory Care, and is made to toe the mark. The same institution may receive millions of Medicaid dollars and be required to meet few, if any, standards. There certainly are no contract requirements and no community advisory board. Yet the legal sanctions for the City Health Department's quality control powers under Medicaid rest on a firm legal foundation while the situation, as we have seen, is quite the opposite for the ACP.

THE ACP AND THE MUNICIPAL HOSPITALS

A major struggle which has enlivened the history of the ACP since its inception has been the attempt by a coalition of city political and health officials and certain citywide consumer-representative groups, such as the Citizens' Committee for Children, to persuade the state government to allow Ghetto Medicine funds to be used to subsidize ambulatory services in municipal as well as voluntary hospitals (Bernstein). Nothing has changed since Bernstein wrote her paper in 1971. The state has continued to reject the proposition, and a change in administration in 1974 made no difference.

Although the work of Betty Bernstein (1971) and others (*Public Health Notes*, 1974) attempts to elevate the matter to a plane of high principle, it appears as if the struggle all boils down to something very simple: money. The state simply does not want to get into the business of further subsidization of the city's hospital system. Those who want Ghetto Medicine money funneled to municipal hospitals continually point to one aspect of the original aim of the program: improvement of health services in underserved areas. However, it must not be forgotten that that aim was conceived of in terms of free-standing health centers, not hospital ambulatory services, and that the use of money to support hospital services at all rests on a very wobbly legal base.

Partisans of support for the municipal hospital system sometimes talk in a way that makes it appear as if they think there is something inherently evil, or at least menacing, in the voluntary hospital system, particularly when it is contrasted with the municipal hospital system. What should be realized is how closely intertwined the two systems are. Many of the larger voluntaries are now serving populations which are virtually indistinguishable from those served by municipal hospitals. Many of the municipal hospitals are staffed with physicians hired under contract for them by voluntary hospitals and medical schools. An increasing amount of the financial support for the voluntaries comes from tax dollars. Boards of Trustees of voluntaries are often seen in certain quarters as malevolent and unsympathetic to the needs of patients, particularly poor ones. But are they any more or less malevolent than the large, cumbersome bureaucracy which operates the municipal hospital system, a system whose historical roots lie in the poor law system? How different are the social class backgrounds and living styles of hospital boards of trustees than those of the Board of Directors of the Health and Hospitals Corporation and of the top officials who run the hospitals? It would be an interesting question to examine. The differences might turn out to be more apparent than real. In reality then, the two systems are at least as much alike as they are different. It is our view that the struggle over the use of Ghetto Medicine funds for municipal hospitals does not properly turn on questions of principle, but only on questions of money.

Ghetto Medicine in Suffolk County

The Suffolk County Ghetto Medicine program is an example of what happened when an attempt was made to implement the program as it was originally conceived, using the allowed contract mechanism. The experience demonstrates the kinds of difficulties which can be encountered when inexperienced county health departments and governments get involved in attempting to develop and operate general ambulatory care services. The major problems which have been encountered, and which continue to be encountered, in making these programs work have been with the county health department and the county government: enormous delays, lack of understanding, conflicts with the civil service system, the county insistence on running pieces of the program itself even when contracting with hospitals to run the bulk of the programs. All of this goes under the heading of "red tape and bureaucracy." We do not know what the experience has been in the other five counties in the state outside of New York City which have Ghetto Medicine programs, but in Suffolk, at least, "red tape and bureaucracy" abound and make program implementation slow and frustrating. That the part of the whole Ghetto Medicine philosophy which puts reliance on county government—not traditionally bastions of innovation and imagination—for its implementation may be basically flawed is indicated by the fact that only about 10 percent of New York State's counties have tried to do anything with it at all.

The community role in Suffolk is very different from that in New York City. A major reason for this is related to the major differences in the roles of the two health departments. In the city, the department clearly has two roles: money-provider and inspector. In Suffolk, at least in those centers operated under contract which we examined, the department's role is muddled. On the one hand, it is the money-giver. On the other hand, however, it has insisted on being, in part, program operator as well. It has its own public health nurses, on its own payroll, under its own supervision, working in direct patient care services in the centers. It owns or leases the buildings, maintains them, and purchases the equipment itself. It runs the family planning and dental services itself. The county's Department of Transportation runs transport services, if any. Yet another agency, the Economic Opportunity Commission, runs the outreach programs. Thus in dealing with the county, the community must relate to part of the program administration as well as to the money-giver. Since, as program-operator the county appears to have severe problems, bordering on the inept, the community groups often find themselves in an adversary position with the county. This is in sharp contrast to the New York City situation in which the Health Department's role is clear, and the department and the Community Board most often find themselves as allies in attempting to improve the various service programs in the hospitals.

Another dimension of this confused role for the county is what it does to the relationship between the contracting institution and the county. In the city, the relationship is again clear. The hospitals have complete operational responsibility. They must deal with the city for money and they must deal with city inspection policies. In

Suffolk County, the contractees must deal with the county as a co-program-operator, as well, in a situation in which the mode in which the county carries out its operational responsibilities often inhibits the contractee's ability to put forward its own best effort.

The bipartite county role also relates, or would appear to relate, to the limited evaluation program which the county has undertaken. It stands in sharp contrast to that of New York City. Part of the reason for the county's practically nonexistent program is related to inexperience, lack of expertise, and its apparent lack of interest in attempting to get outside expert assistance in setting up a program. Part of it also relates, however, directly to the fact that the county is, in part, program-operator. The contradictions involved in being one's own inspector are apparent, and community representatives, well intentioned as they may be, simply lack the sophistication, so evident in New York City, to be able to deal with the situation.

Finally, the Suffolk County Ghetto Medicine experience must give serious pause to those who think that the solutions to all, or even some, of the problems with the health care delivery system in the United States lie in turning over any significant responsibilities for program operations to local governments, at least as they are now presently organized. Even in New York City, which has the most sophisticated and experienced local government in the country, the problems which the government has in health services operations are, as is well known, severe. County governments, at least on the basis of this one example, would appear to be even less well suited to health services operations.

References

Alexander, R. S. Medicaid in New York II: Administrative dynamics in megalopolitan health care. *American Journal of Public Health,* 1969, 59, 815.

Bellin, L. E. Medicaid in New York. III: Utopianism and bare knuckles in public health. Realpolitik in the health care arena—Standard setting of professional services. *American Journal of Public Health,* 1969, 59, 820.

Bellin, L. E., & Kavaler, F. *Policing publicly funded health care for poor quality, overutilization, and fraud: The New York City Medicaid experience.* Paper presented at the annual meeting, American Public Health Association, Philadelphia, Nov. 11, 1969.

Bernstein, B. What happened to "Ghetto medicine" in New York State. *American Journal of Public Health,* 1971, *61,* 1287; see also relevant letters 1972, *62,* 3.

The Joint commission on accreditation of hospitals filed suit. Hospital Week, June 6, 1975, *11* (23).

Jonas, S. A theoretical approach to the question of community control of health services facilities. *American Journal of Public Health,* 1971, *61,* 916.

Kavaler, F. Medicaid in New York. IV: People, providers and payment—Telling it how it is. *American Journal of Public Health,* 1969, *59,* 825.

Medicaid in city scored in audit. *New York Times,* August 4, 1971.

Medicaid audits cited by the city. *New York Times,* January 9, 1972.

City, state and U.S. study abuses in Medicaid here. *New York Times,* Apr. 19, 1975.

O'Rourke, E. Medicaid in New York. I: Introduction. *American Journal of Public Health,* 1969, *59,* 814.

PHANYC urges changes in "Ghetto medicine" program [editorial]. *Public Health Notes,* November 1974, *2,* (20).

9

Lessons from the Study and Implications for National Health Insurance

Introduction

Our study was concerned with the coincidence of two of the major problem areas of the United States health care delivery system: the measurement and regulation of the quality of health care and the delivery of health services in organized ambulatory settings. We examined parts of the operation of two programs of the New York State Department of Health. The first, which is known generically as "Article 28," but which in fact is based on other articles of the State Public Health Laws as well, is concerned with the regulation of hospital operations throughout the state. We examined some of the available material concerning Article 28 operations in general, and gathered information in the field on activities under its provisions directly. The second is known generically as Ghetto Medicine, although there is in fact no single law bearing that name, nor is there a law which describes the program. We looked in some detail at the implementation of a variation upon the original intent of this program in New York City, under the aegis of the New York City Health Department.

Objectively and rationally, quality control and organized ambulatory care are two areas which should receive a great deal of stress in a health care system. For a variety of reasons, in the United States health care delivery system neither has received much attention other than that of the rhetorical variety, although the degree of attention paid has been increasing in recent years. We have, in

128

essence, studied two orphans, two third-rankers, two misfits, and have tried to see, in a certain context, how they have made out when thrown together. From our point of view, which sees the third-class status of quality control and organized ambulatory as a bad thing, some of the observed experience has been good. Some of it has been bad. However, it is possible to learn positive lessons from both good and bad experiences. We feel that we have done so.

Major Lessons

In a study of this size there are obviously many findings, of varying degrees of importance. We do not intend here to review them all, but to concentrate on summarizing the ones which we feel are the most important.

1. *"It doesn't matter how many teeth you have if you can't close your mouth."*

In dealing with the problems of enforcement agencies, some people are wont to say that "the only thing we [they] need is more teeth." Some New York State Health Department officials talked this way in discussing the problems of Article 28. "What we need is one more power," or teeth, they would say. But it is quite obvious that the State Health Department does not, or cannot, use the powers which it already has. It has the teeth, but for a variety of reasons, only some of which are entirely understood, it cannot close its mouth.

As we have said several times, the contrast with what the New York City Health Department has done with the ACP is striking. In the law, the City Health Department has a few teeth. As we have pointed out, the gum structure is very weak, and objectively the teeth are very wobbly. In fact, one well aimed blow could probably knock them out. Again for a variety of reasons, not all of which are well understood, the City Health Department closes its mouth hard, and the few wobbly teeth appear to leave their mark. Not wanting to carry the metaphor any further, we shall consider the point made. To coin a phrase, where there is a will, there is (often although not always) a way.

2. The ACP has been a success.

On the basis of the descriptive evaluations which we heard from hospital directors, hospital directors of ambulatory care, City Health Department officials, and community representatives, the ACP must be considered a success. However, there are limitations. Most of the observers are using implicit criteria only. That is, "does the program match up with what I think is good, without spelling out specific standards?" Even in the few cases where explicit criteria are used—that is, specific standards are set out—they are fairly rough, and correspondingly, the measurements are not terribly precise. Nevertheless, the overwhelmingly positive appraisals must be recognized, even taking the limitations into account. The ACP seems to have had a positive effect on ambulatory care in the participating voluntary hospitals.

3. The key ingredients of the ACP are three.

The ACP has many features. Three of them stand out: money attached to standards; the contract mechanism; the community role in contract enforcement. It needs all three, however, to make it work. That can be understood simply by comparing the ACP with the other programs under which the city government gives money to voluntary hospitals for providing services. Under the Medicaid program, the city's voluntary hospitals receive amounts of money far greater than the amounts received under the ACP. There are Medicaid performance standards. So there is money attached to standards. But there is no contract; Medicaid monies are paid out on a cost-reimbursement basis. There is no community input to standards enforcement. And, for whatever reasons, there is little or no enforcement of standards for institutions under Medicaid in New York City.

The City Health and Hospitals Corporation contracts with voluntary hospitals and medical schools to supply medical staff and certain other services for most of the city hospitals. There is money attached to standards, and there is a contract. There is little or no community input to contract enforcement. Contract enforcement under the so-called Affiliation Agreements is reputed to be weak, for whatever reasons.

Here, then, are two instances in which there are money and standards and, in one of them, a contract, and little or no enforcement. On the other hand, one should not think that the magic answer is the community input alone. In New York City, there have been many instances in which there were very high levels of community input, particularly in the neighborhood health center movement, in which program output left much to be desired in terms of both quality and quantity. The secret of the success of the ACP, is in its melding of the elements. Which leads us to the next point.

4. *The approach of the ACP to community participation is innovative and productive.*

As we pointed out, we did little evaluation of the process of community input to the ACP. However, the outcome looked good. As far as we could tell, the "who is in charge here" questions which bedeviled the neighborhood health center movement, particularly that of the Office of Economic Opportunity, have been left behind in the ACP. The community representatives' principal role is clear: contract negotiator, and contract enforcer to both the contractor and the contractee. This, to use an overused word, is *meaningful* community participation. In other words, it is *productive*.

5. *The original concept of ghetto medicine has its problems.*

We looked at the program of only one of the six counties outside of New York City which have tried to implement Ghetto Medicine. We do not know if Suffolk County's experience is typical. However, the reviews of the program in Suffolk County are, at best, mixed. The health center programs are of uncertain quality and produce a rather low volume of service. The county was already pledged to undertake a program of developing neighborhood health centers. It is impossible to determine whether or not the Ghetto Medicine program helped, hindered, or altered in any way the development of that program. Suffolk County chose to use the contract mechanism for its program, but in actuality the programs are run by (and suffer severely with) a combined county-contractee administrative mechanism. One thing that the experience shows very clearly is the tremendous limitations which county government has in trying to implement an innovative program. If the Suffolk County experience is any indication, county government is not the instrument which would be one's first choice to do something new, regardless of the reasons for their limitations. That county government was chosen as the lynchpin for the original program was one of the major reasons for the almost complete failure of Ghetto Medicine, as it originally appeared on the statute books, to alter the profile of health care in New York State.

6. *Article 28 is selectively enforced.*

It is obvious that Article 28 has had no effect, positive or negative, on hospital ambulatory care in New York State, because the relevant sections of the Hospital Code written pursuant to it have never been enforced. No one, of course, has any idea what might happen if the code were to be enforced, but, as we have pointed out, structural standards have their limitations. Beyond the limited area of hospital ambulatory care standards, the overall effects of Article 28 remain virtually unevaluated with the exception of one retrospective statistical study of certification-of-need. A factor in this selectivity may be the virtual lack of public involvement in its work. In one area of its Article 28 activities, the nursing home industry, the State Health Department has recently shown itself responsive to public pressure, and has also shown that it can benefit in carrying out its responsibilities from public support.

7. *The New York State Health Department does not use all of its powers.*

We can elaborate little upon this statement, because we did not look into the "why's." But even without understanding them, the fact is useful to know.

8. *The voluntary hospital system has potential for positive change.*

It is popular in some quarters to seek the solution to the problems faced by the American health care system in a "government takeover" of that system. The results of this study can be used in response to that argument. The voluntary hospitals which participate in the program have shown themselves to be capable of positive change. It is true that in many cases change is made with great reluctance and may be, at this early stage, more apparent than real. Furthermore, changes, in terms of program, approach to community participation, and approach to quality control, are being made only for the stepchild, ambulatory care. The hospitals are still playing overprotective mothers to their prides and joys, the inpatient services. But history moves only one step at a time, except in revolutionary situations. Change has begun, and the voluntaries are participating, or, as some might put it, being forced to participate.

On the other hand, government as a program operator doesn't come off too well in the one instance in which we looked at it in depth. However, going farther afield than the efforts of one medium-large county in a neighborhood health center program (just imagine smaller counties trying to do something), do we really want our hospital system to look like that of the Health and Hospital Corporation of New York City or of the Veterans' Administration? For a variety of reasons, government efforts in health care delivery in this country have been for categories of people (the federal level), categories of diseases (the state level), or categories of socioeconomic class (the local level). This history binds American government as it is presently constituted to certain attitudes and limited capabilities as a direct deliverer of care. It would appear that the results of our study lend some credence to the view that the voluntary hospital system, forced to become publicly accountable and responsive to the broad mass of the people which it serves, is reasonably well equipped to undertake the necessary changes in our health care system, to the extent positive change is possible within the limits of our present socioeconomic system.

9. *There is a yawning chasm between the academic and operational communities concerned with quality of medical care.*

The academics and the operational people in quality of medical care just do not seem to communicate. The literature, by and large, does not address itself to the real world faced, say, by a state health department in trying to implement a hospital licensing law. Perhaps that is one reason why health department personnel don't seem to be too familiar with the quality of care literature.

This situation leads to some disastrous results. The academic literature has to all intents and purposes concluded that structural standards have no validity in auditing the quality of medical care. On the operational side, however, most official agencies involved in quality of care regulation, with the exception of PSROs, rely almost exclusively on structural techniques. (The New York City Health Department is one exception to this rule, using process as well as structural techniques in the ACP.) Nevertheless, the academic community does little research into the problem area of the practical difficulties of actually implementing valid and reliable quality measurement and control programs. It should be noted that not only do academics virtually ignore official agencies, but they provide little practical guidance for hospital medical staff review committees as well.

10. *Full evaluation of the present operational quality measurement and control systems and of operational planning systems is needed.*

It is not known what the effects of Article 28 and programs like it really are. Yet the country plunges ahead, legislating like mad. This is likely our most important finding.

Recommendations

On the basis of the ten lessons and other lesser conclusions discussed ad seriatim in the report, we came up with a series of recommendations. Most of them are for experimentation and further study. Although the ACP comes up smelling like a rose and Article 28 implementation, especially in hospital ambulatory care, doesn't look too good, we were most impressed with the extent of our findings concerning what is poorly understood or simply not known.

1. The Article 28 experience should be fully evaluated on two levels. First, the extent to which all of the provisions of Article 28 and the codes written pursuant to it have been and are being actually implemented should be determined. Second, the meaning and utility of Article 28 and its codes for the quality of medical care should be determined.

2. Studies should be made of similar efforts in other states.

3. The ACP should be evaluated using objective, statistical measures of performance. Has the ACP really made the difference most people think it has? If so, are the key elements really the contract, the money and the community? The whole current process of community participation in the ACP should be evaluated since the one comprehensive study was made in 1971 and the program has changed a great deal.

4. The whole area of public accountability in health services deserves some careful attention. This would include public accountability of institutional and individual providers, of public bodies (i.e., regional planning boards), and government agencies. Such studies would consider also the question of the utility and productivity of public accountability.

5. The implications for Professional Standards Review Organizations of our findings concerning medical care quality control measures, particularly in the areas of methodology and public accountability, should be explored.

6. We recommend that efforts be made to develop educational and technical assistance programs under Article 28, Ghetto Medicine, and similar programs. We believe that it is important for operational quality control programs to move beyond policing and inspecting to educating and improving, except where policing is entirely appropriate, as in the proprietary nursing home industry. In the ACP in particular, a creative approach would be the introduction of peer participation in inspection and of self-evaluation in the review process.

7. Explorations must be undertaken concerning the mechanisms through which the academic and operational quality-of-medical-care communities can be brought together, at least to some extent. One approach might be to broaden and stiffen the evaluation of academic health science institutions themselves. They are now virtually immune to both government and public scrutiny, subject only to very closed, private accreditation processes. Change there could be very healthy, for many reasons.

Implications for National Health Insurance

Virtually all of the lessons which we drew from our study have implications for any national health insurance program which might be established in the United States. However, there is one which stands out above all of the others in its importance and potential impact: the utility of the contract method in disbursing government funds to private providers of health services. Elsewhere (Jonas, 1974, 1975) I have argued strongly against including the commercial insurance industry in any national health insurance plan principally because I think that so doing would pave the way for a complete private corporate take-over of the United States health care delivery system. But the contract method of reimbursement could and should be experimented with regardless of the form national health insurance takes.

Presently, reimbursement under the vast majority of third-party payment plans in this country is on an item-of-service basis. Hospitals are reimbursed according to the number of days of care provided, the number of X-rays provided, and so on. Doctors are reimbursed for the number of visits made, the number of operations performed, and the like. Quantity of work, but not necessarily quality of work in either individual or community terms, is rewarded under our present approach.

The contract mechanism appears to hold great promise for improvement of care in a number of areas. Among them are cost control, medical quality, geographic distribution, and specialty distribution. On the basis of the experience with the ACP, it appears as if there are two key elements in making the contract mechanism a success, in addition to money and a provider willing to operate on a contract basis. One is a contractor capable of devising a workable program, and of carrying out inspections with some degree of efficiency, expertise, and objectivity. The other is a third party, representing the users of the service for which the contract is made, which can effectively participate in contract negotiation and enforcement.

Contracts for a whole package of services, inpatient and outpatient, could be made between a national health insurance agency and a hospital. A formula could be worked out to peg payment to a combination of cost, volume of service, and quality of care, with rewards for good service and penalties for bad service. The criteria of performance would be much more complex for a whole hospital than for an ambulatory service alone, of course. The devising of a fair contract with a reasonable payment formula and a workable inspection plan would be very difficult, to be sure. However, if a small understaffed bureau in a local health department beset by continual shrinkage of its financial base could do as creative a job as it did, I strongly believe that the technical problems could be solved. The contract mechanism could even be applied to individual physicians working in their own offices, provided they were paid by salary or capitation.

Ever increasing amounts of public money are being spent in the health care delivery system. In the mid-sixties the government share was about 25 percent of the total. In the mid-seventies, the figure was 40 percent. By the mid-eighties, it is likely to be in the 75 percent range. The contract approach would for the first time give the payers, that is the people, some real control over what the providers are doing, aside from the malpractice litigation route which is properly used only in extreme cases of poor care, and dependence on the professional integrity of the providers. Utilization review in Medicare and fraud controls in Medicaid have not been especially effective in assuring that the public's personal health service dollars have been well spent. PSRO may bring about some improvements, especially in the area of technical, medical quality, which is certainly important. But PSRO is based on peer review, which has its limitations. The contract mechanism takes a big step forward, providing for real, meaningful public participation in the health care delivery system.

Facing all of the problems which we now have, with an array of possible solutions which themselves have many limitations, I feel that, at least on an experimental basis, under national health insurance, we should try out the contract mechanism of paying for health services.

References

Jonas, S. Issues in national health insurance in the United States of America. *Lancet*, July 20, 1974, p. 143.

Jonas, S. *The economy and health care policy: The corporatization of American medical practice.* Paper delivered at the annual meeting of the American Public Health Association, Chicago, November 17, 1975.

APPENDIX 1

List of Appendixes from Original Report

I. List of Interviewees
II. List of Documents Reviewed
III. New York State Public Health Laws
IV. New York State Health Code
V. Ghetto Medicine Documents:
    1A. The New York Health Center Bill, 1919
    1B. Chapter 662, L. 1923
    2A. Andrew Fleck statement: "Health Services for the Disadvantaged"
    2B. Andrew Fleck letter to Lyons, July 6, 1967
    3. Chapter 572, L. 1968
    4. Announcement by Governor Nelson Rockefeller, June 17, 1968
    5. Chapter 967, L. 1968, with Governor Rockefeller's statement
    6. Chapter 35, L. 1969
    7. State Aid Manual
    8. Governor Rockefeller's announcement, November 6, 1969
    9. First "Ghetto Medicine" contract prototype
    10. First draft, New York City Ghetto Medicine "Guidelines," April 29, 1971
    11. Second draft, New York City Ghetto Medicine "Guidelines"
    12. 1974-75 Ambulatory Care Program contract
    13. Ambulatory Care Program contract schedules
    14. Evaluation Process in Ambulatory Care, 1971
    15A. Evaluation Process in Ambulatory Care, 1975
    15B. New York City Department of Health Audit Form
    16. Site Visit Reports, Methodist Hospital, Brooklyn, N.Y., 1974 and 1975

APPENDIX 2

List of Interviewees

Bellin, L. E.   Commissioner of Health, New York City Department of Health

Bernstein, B.   Associate Director, Citizens' Committee for Children, New York, N.Y.

Bernstein, G.   Formerly Assistant Commissioner, New York City Department of Health, presently Director of Development, Church Charity Foundation, Brooklyn, N.Y.

Borsody, R.   Attorney. New York, N.Y.

Brickner, P. W.   Acting Director, Department of Community Medicine, Saint Vincent's Hospital, New York, N.Y.

Ciccro, F.   Deputy Commissioner, New York State Department of Health

Fearon, Z.   Chairperson, Consumer Council to the [City] Health Department, New York, N.Y.

Fleck, A.   Assistant Commissioner, formerly First Deputy Commissioner, New York State Department of Health

Freiwirth, M.   Executive Director, Mary Immaculate Hospital, Queens, N.Y.

Gambuti, G.   Executive Vice-President, Saint Luke's Hospital, New York, N.Y.

Garry, J.   Director, Bureau of Ambulatory Care, New York State Department of Health

141

Gentry, J.   Director, Bureau of Health Care Services, New York City Department of Health

Gitman, L.   Director, Division of Patient Care Services, Department of Health Services, Suffolk County, N.Y.

Hammerling, A.   Assistant Vice-President for Ambulatory Care Services, Roosevelt Hospital, New York, N.Y.

Harris, D.   Associate Director, Mount Sinai Hospital, New York, N.Y.

Hong, J.   Director of Ambulatory Care, Mary Immaculate Hospital, Queens, N.Y.

McLaughlin, M.   Commissioner, Department of Health Services, Suffolk County, N.Y.

Mazzola, G.   Department of Community Medicine, Brookhaven Memorial Hospital, Patchogue, N.Y.

Metsch, J. M.   Assistant Professor, Program in Health Care Administration, City University of New York

Miller, H.   Chairman, New York State Assembly Health Committee

Neiman, S.   Director of Community Medicine, Methodist Hospital, Brooklyn, N.Y.

O'Connor, W.   Director, Martin Luther King Health Center, Wyandanch, N.Y.

Pomrinse, S. D.   Director, Mount Sinai Hospital and Medical Center, New York, N.Y.

Reichman, S.   Director of Community Medicine, Hospital for Joint Diseases, New York, N.Y.

Ruben, D.   Director, Consumer Commission on the Accreditation of Health Services, New York, N.Y.

Schrager, W.   Health and Hospital Planning Council of Southern New York

Schwarz, A.   Assistant Commissioner for Evaluation and Institutional Review, New York City Department of Health

Shapiro, M. B.   Director, Bureau of Economic Analysis, New York State Department of Health

Solomon, D.   Director, Hospital Construction Finance, New York State Health Department

Terenzio, J. V.   President, United Hospital Fund, New York, N.Y.

Travers, T.   New York City Department of Health

Urquhart, B.   Division of Patient Care Services, Department of Health Services, Suffolk County, N.Y.

Wainfeld, B.   Director of Community Medicine, Brookdale Hospital, Brooklyn, N.Y.

Wynne, J.   Comptroller, Mary Immaculate Hospital, Queens, N.Y.

Public Health Laws, New York State:
Summary of Pertinent Sections

1. *Public Health Law*

    a. *Article 2*

    *Sec. 201 details the "functions, powers and duties of the department." Interestingly enough, the Article 28 powers are not specifically referred to in this section.

    *Sec. 206 describes the "Commissioner; general powers and duties."
    The Commissioner shall: (a) take cognizance of the interests of health and life of the people of the state, and of all matters pertaining thereto and exercise the functions, powers and duties of the department prescribed by law: . . . (j) cause to be made such scientific studies and research which have for their purpose the reduction of morbidity and mortality and the improvement of the quality of medical care through the conduction of medical audits within the state. . . .

    These wide powers are just a selection of those conferred upon the Commissioner.

    *Sec. 220 establishes the Public Health Council.

    *Sec. 225 describes the duties of the Council. Among them are:
    1. The public health council shall, at the request of the Commissioner, consider any matter relating to the preservation and improvement of public health, and may advise the commissioner thereon; and it may, from time to time, submit to the commissioner, any recommendations relating to the preservation and improvement of public health. . . .
    4. The sanitary code may:
    (a) deal with any matters affecting the security of life or health

or the preservation and improvement of public health in the state of New York, and with any matters as to which the jurisdiction is conferred upon the public health council; . . .

The balance of the powers deal with the Sanitary Code.

b. *Article 28*

*Sec. 2800 is the "Declaration of policy and statement of purpose."
Hospital and related services including health-related service of the highest quality, efficiently provided and properly utilized at a reasonable cost, are of vital concern to the public health. In order to provide for the protection and promotion of the health of the inhabitants of the state, pursuant to section three of the article seventeen of the state constitution, the department of health shall have the central, comprehensive responsibility for the development and administration of the state's policy with respect to hospital and related services, and all public and private institutions, whether state, county, municipal, incorporated or not incorporated, serving principally as facilities for the prevention, diagnosis or treatment of human disease, pain, injury, deformity or physical conditions or for the rendering of health-related service shall be subject to the provisions of this article.

*Sec. 2801 contains the important definitions.

*Sec. 2801–a concerns "Establishment or incorporation of hospitals," conferring final authority to do so upon the Public Health Council.

*Sec. 2802. "Approval of construction." Despite the very broad powers in reference to hospital "establishment or incorporation" conferred upon the Public Health Council in Sec. 2801–a, this section confers specific powers over construction upon the Commissioner, to wit: "The construction of a hospital, whether public or private, incorporated or not incorporated, shall require the prior approval of the commissioner."

*Sec. 2803 "Commissioner and council; powers and duties." ("Council" here refers to the Public Health Council.)
1. The commissioner shall have the power to inquire into the

operation of hospitals and to conduct periodic inspections of facilities with respect to the fitness and adequacy of the premises, equipment, personnel, rules and by-laws, standards of medical care, hospital service, including health-related service system of accounts, records, and the adequacy of financial resources and sources of future revenues.

2. The council, by a majority vote of its members, shall adopt and amend rules and regulations, subject to the approval of the commissioner, to effectuate the provisions and purposes of this article, including, but not limited to (a) the establishment of requirements for a uniform statewide system of reports and audits relating to the quality of medical and physical care provided, hospital utilization and costs, (b) establishment by the department of schedules of rates, payments, reimbursements, grants and other charges for hospital and health-related services as provided in section two thousand eight hundred and seven, (c) standards and procedures relating to hospital operating certificates, and (d) the establishment of a system of accounts and cost finding for each class. The commissioner may propose rules and regulations and amendments thereto for consideration by the council. . . .

4. At the request of the commissioner, hospitals shall furnish to the department such reports and information as it may require to effectuate the provisions of this article. . . .

Very broad powers in reference to measuring and regulating the quality of medical care are granted to both the Commissioner and the Public Health Council by this section.

*Sec. 2805 requires hospitals to have Operating Certificates, (licenses).

*Sec. 2806 deals with suspension or revocation of a Hospital Operating Certificate. It states in part:

1. A hospital operating certificate may be revoked, suspended, limited, or annulled by the commissioner or the health services administration of the city of New York, as the case may be, on proof that: (a) the hospital has failed to comply with the provisions of this article or rules and regulations promulgated thereunder. . . .

*Sec. 2807 deals with the rate-setting powers.

c. *Article 29*: "Hospital Survey, Planning, and Review."

*Sec. 2901 elaborates the functions of the Department in relation to hospital planning, although Sec. 2802 clearly gives the Commissioner final authority over construction.

*Sec. 2903 places control over the Hill-Burton program or any successor in the hands of the Health Department.

*Sec. 2904 defines the hospital review and planning councils.

Hospital Code of New York State:
Summary of Pertinent Sections

The Hospital Code is one portion, Part 700, of the State Health Code, known officially as the "Official Compilation, Codes, Rules and Regulations of the State of New York, 10, Health (A.B.C.)."

*Section 700.2 contains all of the relevant definitions.

*Part 701 is concerned with Operating Certificates. The very detailed requirements are based upon the powers granted to the Public Health Council by Article 28, Section 2803.

*Section 701.3 details the types of changes in hospitals for which Departmental approval is required.

*Part 703 sets the basic standards for Ambulatory Services. This is part of the "General Provisions," Subchapter A of the Hospital Code. The most important portions (see also Appendix 7) are:

*"Section 703.1 Applicability. The provisions of this Part shall apply to hospitals with outpatient departments and to independent out-of-hospital health facilities which accept primary responsibility for health supervision and medical care of patients. . . .

*"703.3 Medical service plan. Facilities providing ambulatory services shall submit to the department a plan governing the provision of medical services to patients, which has been approved by the governing authority and the medical staff, including, as a minimum, the following:
  (a) a comprehensive medical evaluation for such patients on a periodic basis . . .
  (b) continuity of care . . .
  (c) the method of scheduling patient visits to physicians with general scheduling of not more than five patients per hour with an allowance of at least 30 minutes for the first complete patient workup . . .

148

°"703.4 Extension clinics. Notwithstanding the requirements of this Chapter, extension clinics of hospitals with outpatient departments and of independent out-of-hospital health facilities shall submit to the department a plan acceptable to the commissioner governing the location and objectives of the extension clinic, the relationships to the parent organization and a detailed program of operation."

°Parts 710 and 711 set the detailed standards for medical facility construction.

°Part 720 sets the standards for the "Organization and Administration" of hospitals. These are part of Subchapter C of the Hospital Code, "Hospital Operation." They are much more detailed standards for operation than are found in Part 703 of Subchapter A, "General Provisions." The Sections of Part 720 dealing with ambulatory services are summarized here.

°Section 720.17 concerns Emergency departments. Parts (a) and (b) deal with physician staffing. Part (c) deals with nurse staffing. Part (d) concerns nursing personnel education in emergency services. Part (e) lists required equipment, in quite a bit of detail, even to describing the contents of various surgical trays. Part (f) lists the items or classes of items of drugs and biologicals which shall be immediately available. Part (g) requires lists of standard equipment and supplies to be compiled and posted. Part (h) requires an emergency department procedure manual. Part (i) lists the required minimum medical, surgical and ancillary services. Part (j) states the requirements for emergency room records. Parts (k) through (n) contain other miscellaneous requirements.

°Section 720.18 concerns outpatient departments. Part (a) states that: "all applicable policies pertaining to the organization and administration of the hospital, including the medical staff, shall also apply to the outpatient department." Part (b) lists basic requirements for outpatient department services:

(1) provide such diagnostic and therapeutic services for medical diagnosis, treatment and preventive care of well and injured or sick persons by means of organized sessions or clinics, the number

and frequency of such clinic sessions being determined by the needs of the patients for whom it accepts responsibility;

(2) provide for comprehensive medical evaluation of all new patients registered in the clinic, unless satisfactory record of such examination made within the previous six months is made part of the medical record within 30 days after registration;

(3) include provisions acceptable to the commissioner pertaining to standards of medical care of ambulatory patients in the by-laws, rules and regulations of the hospital and the medical staff;

(4) provide an organized medical staff which may include doctors of medicine, osteopathy, and dentistry; and

(5) have on the premises or have access to approved laboratory and radiology services."

Parts (c) through (h) deal with outpatient department personnel requirements, including those for physicians. Part (i) concerns medical records. Part (j) covers outpatient surgical procedures. Part (k) covers requirements for social services. Part (1) concerns the pharmacy.

APPENDIX 5

The New York Health Center Bill

Memorandum as to the provisions of a bill authorizing a county, city, or consolidated health district to create and maintain one or more health centers and providing State aid therefor.

Prepared by the Public Health Council and Recommended by the Commissioner of Health. Fortieth Annual Report of the New York State Department of Health for the Year ending December 31, 1919, pp. 7–11.

PURPOSES

1. To provide for the residents of rural districts, for industrial workers and all others in need of such service, scientific medical and surgical treatment, hospital and dispensary facilities, and nursing care, at a cost within their means or, if necessary, free.

2. To assist the local medical practitioners by providing:

(a) Facilities for accurate diagnosis by a coordinated group of specially qualified physicians and surgeons, both for hospital patients and for outpatients.

(b) Consultation and advice as to treatment by medical and surgical experts.

(c) Clinical, bacteriological and chemical laboratory service and X-ray facilities at moderate cost or free when necessary.

3. To encourage and provide facilities for an annual medical examination to detect physical defects and disease, and to discover conditions favorable to the development of disease, and to indicate methods of correcting the same.

4. To provide or aid in securing adequate school medical inspection and school nursing service.

5. To secure or aid in securing better enforcement of the Public Health Law and a more effective administration of Public Health activities within the area served.

6. To provide a Public Health nursing service adapted to and adequate for the community served.

7. To aid in securing the dissemination of information in regard to Public Health throughout the area served.

151

8. To aid in securing adequate compensation for medical and surgical care rendered in hospitals and clinics, in order that efficient service may be everywhere available.

9. To provide laboratories, group diagnosticians, consultants and hospital facilities in the smaller cities and rural districts, and to counteract the growing tendency of medical practitioners to remove to larger centers, and to attract to and to retain in the practice of medicine in these communities a large number of qualified practitioners of both sexes.

10. To provide medical libraries including books, pamphlets, periodic leaflets, exhibits, moving-picture films, and kindred educational facilities with halls for meetings if needed.

11. To provide hospital and other necessary resources for dealing promptly with epidemics.

12. To reduce illness and disability among the industrial workers of the State by providing prompt and accurate diagnosis and efficient treatment for sick and injured workers and the members of their families.

13. To coordinate Public Health activities within the districts.

HEALTH CENTERS

1. A health center may consist of the following parts, any one or more of which parts may be established at one time with the approval of the State Commissioner of Health and the formulation of a general plan for the whole center.

(a) Hospitals: The erection of new hospitals or arrangements with other institutions, or both, so that they shall form essential parts of the center. Such hospitals may include as units thereof existing or hereafter established hospitals or pavilions for the care of tuberculosis, for cases of other communicable disease, for children, for cases of maternity and mental diseases and for other groups. Existing tuberculosis hospitals may become parts of the health center of a city or county by which they may have been established.

(b) Clinics for Out-patients: including especially those now regarded as public health clinics, such as those for tuberculosis, venereal disease, prenatal and child welfare, mental and nervous diseases and defects and clinics for school children, dental clinics, and also medical, surgical and diagnostic clinics.

(c) Clinical, Bacteriological and Chemical Laboratories, auxiliary to the State Laboratory, and X-ray laboratories with services at moderate charges, or free, affording modern laboratory facilities needed in the diagnosis and treatment of disease.

(d) District Health Service with a district health officer and deputy

health officers in various parts of the district, such districts to be either
a city or county, or a consolidation of two or more existing health districts (such consolidation to be approved by the State Commissioner of
Health). The present health officers in these districts shall act as deputies
during their present terms of office. In the subsequent appointments of
deputies in the various portions of the districts, persons residing therein
possessing the qualifications prescribed by the Public Health Council
shall have preference. Each local health board shall appoint for its town
or village a deputy to the health officer of the health center district.

(e) Public Health Nursing Service, including school nursing for all
parts of the district.

(f) Center for School Medical Inspection with proper medical supervision and facilities to enable practitioners to provide adequate treatment
for all school children showing physical defects or disease.

(g) Headquarters for all Health, Medical, Nursing, and other Public
Welfare Activities of the district which wish to utilize the center.

2. The locations, sites, plans and initial equipment of the health center shall be subject to the approval of the State Department of Health.
The State Department of Health and the State Architect shall provide
model plans for such centers for any community requesting them.

STATE AID TO HEALTH CENTERS

1. To be granted for each hospital bed constructed or provided for
under this statute.

(a) For new construction and equipment of hospitals, one-half of
the cost to be paid by the State, such payment not to exceed $750 per
bed, and beds for the purpose of this provision to be in proportion not
in excess of one to each 500 of the population.

(b) A grant of 60 cents per day for every free patient maintained
in any hospital operated as a part of a health center.

2. To be granted for clinics and annual medical examinations.

(a) A grant for the creation of out-patient clinics equal to one-half
of the initial cost of establishment, the amount to be paid by the State
for this purpose not to exceed $5,000 per clinic, and 20 cents for each
free treatment in such clinic; one such center for each district, provided
that in counties or cities or districts having more than 50,000 inhabitants
or major fraction thereof.

(b) A grant of 50 cents for each free comprehensive annual medical
examination made at the health center.

3. For the maintenance of laboratories:

A grant from the State of one-half of the annual cost of maintenance of the laboratory of a health center, the sum to be paid by the State not to exceed $3,000 per annum for each laboratory, and $1,500 toward the initial installation and equipment of such laboratory.

4. For salaries of Deputy Health Officers:

A grant of 10 cents per capita per annum toward the salaries of deputy health officers in health districts having less than 1,500 population, and of 5 cents per capita per annum in health districts having a population between 1,500 and 3,000, in addition to such salaries as they are entitled to receive from the local treasury.

5. The total annual grants for the construction of hospitals and clinics shall not be in excess of $2,000,000. Salaries and travelling expenses of consultants and experts employed by the State Department of Health, and other expenses necessarily incurred by the State Department of Health in the enforcement of this law, shall be paid from the sum appropriated for grants toward maintenance and operation of health centers—this sum not to exceed $250,000 per annum.

The District Health Officer may be the superintendent of the hospital and general director of health of the district and of the hospital and medical activities connected therewith. The qualifications for district health officers, deputy health officers, superintendents of hospitals and medical activities, chiefs of clinics and other medical officials and nurses shall be fixed by the Public Health Council, and their appointments be subject to the regulations of the State Civil Service Commission.

The work of all health centers, hospitals, clinics, district laboratories, etc., connected therewith shall be inspected and standardized by the State Department of Health, and the State grants shall be paid only on the written approval of the State Commissioner of Health.

Provision shall be made for occasional or periodic consultations or clinics at the health centers by specialists in medicine and surgery to be furnished through the State Department of Health, and wide previous public announcement of these clinics and consultations shall be made. At these consultations and clinics, health officers and physicians may bring patients for assistance in diagnosis and for advice as to treatment. Fees received from these consultations for the State service shall be credited to the hospital or center where the service is rendered.

The health center laboratories shall be under the supervision of the Director of the State Health Department Laboratories, in order that their work may be maintained at a high level of efficiency; and the facilities of the State Laboratory service shall be available to supplement those of the laboratories of the health centers.

The salaries of the medical and surgical staff, the fees for medical and surgical care, and the conditions for free service in the hospitals and clinics shall be determined by the Boards of Managers. The method of appointment and the composition of such Boards of Managers of the health centers and hospitals to be provided for in this bill.

Official Compilation Codes, Rules and Regulations
of the State of New York 10 Health (A):
Chapter II Administrative Rules and Regulations,
Limitations of Grants

40.10 Granting of State aid. State aid will be granted as follows:

(a) County or part-county health districts. . . .

(2) The cost of maintaining and operating clinics and programs as follows:

(i) Approved preventive, diagnostic, consultation and detection clinics and programs.

(ii) Approved general medical clinics, subject to the following conditions:

(a) A letter of intent as specified in section 710.2 of the New York State Hospital Code must be transmitted in triplicate to the State Commissioner of Health through the regional health director having jurisdiction for each clinic to be maintained and operated. Such letter must include a justification for the clinic and in the location proposed, description of services to be rendered, description of the facility, and a detailed budget showing positions, salaries, manner of payment for personnel and other costs and anticipated revenues. Changes of program must be submitted to the regional health director.

(b) All applicable provisions of Subchapter F of the State Hospital Code as determined by the commissioner must be substantially met.

(c) A fee schedule must be established and arrangements must be made to collect fees from each patient, or a person or private or public agency responsible for his care. The fee schedule must be based upon an annual cost determination process and is to be approved by the State Commissioner of Health.

(d) A county or part-county health commissioner may, in his discretion, in proper cases, where substantial justice will best be served thereby, waive the collection of such fees or compromise any portion of them if the requisite prior approval of the appropriate county body or officer has been obtained as required by law.

(e) The administration of the clinic shall be under the general supervision of the county health commissioner.

(f) Clinic services may be provided by the contract; such contracts must be reviewed and approved by the State Commissioner of Health prior to becoming effective.

(g) An advisory committee of not less than seven persons, representative of the community served, shall be appointed by the county health commissioner. A majority of the committee shall be made up of persons not directly engaged in the health profession. . . .

(c) Cities with 50,000 or more population according to the last preceding federal census. (1) The cost of operating the city health department, provided that public health projects and personnel shall be under the immediate direction of the qualified full-time city health officer or of a deputy health officer. Vacancies in the position of health officer shall be filled promptly, preferably within six months.

(2) The cost of maintaining and operating clinics and programs as follows:

(i) Approved preventive, diagnostic, consultation and detection clinics and programs.

(ii) Approved general medical clinics, subject to the following conditions: [The text of this article then continues as a verbatim repetition of article 40.10 (a) (2) (ii) cited above]. . . .

Chapter V State Hospital Code
Part 703: Ambulatory Services

[Statutory authority: Public Health Law, 2803 (2803–2c)]

703.3 Medical service plan. Facilities providing ambulatory services shall submit to the department a plan governing the provision of medical services to patients, which has been approved by the governing authority and the medical staff, including, as a minimum, the following:

(a) a comprehensive medical evaluation for such patients on a periodic basis indicating the method of selection of patients for annual or other periodic examination:

(b) continuity of care when such patients require hospitalization, home care or emergency care when such services in the facility are not available;

(c) the method of scheduling patient visits to physicians with general scheduling of not more than five patients per hour with an allowance of at least 30 minutes for the first complete patient workup;

(d) where a specific provision of the plan required cannot be implemented immediately, a plan of implementation shall be included, with the anticipated time limit for achieving each phase of the objective specified; and

(e) where it is deemed necessary that any provision of the plan required should be waived indefinitely because of practical difficulties or unnecessary hardships in complying therewith, where such waiver is in the community interest and does not adversely affect the protection of the health of the patient, a request for such waiver and the reasons therefor.

703.4 Extension clinics. Notwithstanding the requirements of this Chapter, extension clinics of hospitals with outpatient departments and of independent out-of-hospital health facilities shall submit to the department a plan acceptable to the commissioner governing the location and objectives of the extension clinic, the relationships to the parent organization and a detailed program of operation.

APPENDIX 8

Official Compilation Codes, Rules and Regulations of the State of New York 10 Health (A): General Provisions Regarding the Payment of State Aid for the Fiscal Year Beginning April 1, 1974

39.3 Methods of payment. The following methods of payment shall apply to the several State aid Programs: . . .

(d) (1) State aid for the operation of medical clinics. State aid will be based on prior approval of specific local programs, after application by the locality, and review and approval by the State Commissioner of Health. Claims must be submitted quarterly by all jurisdictions not later than two months after the calendar quarter in which the expenditures claimed were made. Upon receipt of the fourth claim from all jurisdictions, or after June 15, 1975, the Commissioner of Health shall calculate the amounts claimed by each claimant during the entire year and shall distribute any balance remaining in the total allocated for the payment of State aid for medical clinics in proportion to the relationship which each claimant's total expenditures bears to the total expenditures of all claimants, except that no claimant shall receive more than 50 percent of its total expense.

(2) Any jurisdiction otherwise eligible for State aid under this section that wishes to participate in the State aid program to relieve deficits in voluntary hospitals related to the provision of ambulatory care through the matching of voluntary contributions in cash, securities or other liquid assets unrelated to the provision of services must present to the Commissioner of Health, for approval, appropriately executed contracts with such hospitals and must meet the following conditions before the Commissioner of Health will grant his approval. . . .

Ghetto Medicine Outpatient Department Guidelines, First Draft, 4/29/71

It is explicit for all hospitals in the Ghetto Medicine Program to strive to render comprehensive health care in their respective outpatient departments, and that this care will be family oriented and wherever possible provided at such times as may be most convenient to the consumers of service.

The hospital shall maintain an outpatient department responsible to the Director of Ambulatory Care who shall devise a mechanism which insures a review of care rendered, the education of outpatient department personnel and the efficient administration of the outpatient department.

The hospital shall devise plans that will allow for the smooth referral from and to the outpatient department to the emergency service and vice versa.

The hospital shall in cooperation with the Director of Ambulatory Care institute ongoing audit and review of these guidelines to determine the degree to which they have been implemented, as well as those aspects which have not been implemented.

ADMISSION TO INPATIENT STATUS

Procedures should be established for the smooth transfers from outpatient to inpatient status. Wherever possible the admitting outpatient officer should be the physician of record on the inpatient service to assure continuity.

APPOINTMENTS

The hospital shall strive to provide a meaningful appointment system, one in which waits for new patients will not exceed three weeks and for revisit patients waits not to exceed two weeks.

INTERPRETER

Interpreters should be readily available to clinic patients and staff when needed.

LABORATORY, X-RAY AND PHARMACY

A professional person, preferably a physician, should be assigned to review all laboratory and X-ray reports in an effort to process all negative lab and X-ray reports properly and assure excellence in follow up.

A professional person, preferably a clinic nurse, should be assigned the responsibility to check on "drugs ordered" in order to eliminate contraindicated drugs and/or excess drugs being ordered.

Lab, X-ray and pharmacy services should be available during the times of clinic operation.

MANUAL

The outpatient department shall develop an administrative procedure manual and submit it to the Department of Health.

NURSING

It is important that the integrity of the nursing service be maintained and that as much as is possible nursing staff should perform nursing duties. One nurse, preferably on non-rotating basis should be designated as the head of each clinic to assure continuity of nursing care.

PHYSICAL PLANT

The physical plant of the outpatient department shall conform to all City and State standards as well as making available to the consumers of service waiting areas that are comfortable and that will afford the dignity to which he is entitled.

PHYSICIAN STAFFING

Staffing of physicians will be in comformity to State and City law. Number of assigned physicians will be determined by the activity of a particular clinic.

Physician scheduling should be in conformity with philosophy of continuity of care which will result in returning patients being seen by their original physician whenever possible.

RECORDS

A unit record should be kept incorporating the inpatient, outpatient and emergency services information. Records should be available to the physician at the time of the clinic session and to the nursing staff 12 hours prior to the clinic session.

SOCIAL WORK

A senior social work supervisor should be assigned under the joint supervision of the Department of Social Services and the Director of Ambulatory Care. The function of this worker would be the coordination and liaison between social service staff and the department.

Social workers should be assigned to be physically present at all "major" clinic sessions and be on call to subspecialty clinics. In no case should patient waiting time for social worker exceed one hour.

DIRECTOR OF AMBULATORY CARE

The Director of Ambulatory Care shall be in charge of the outpatient department and shall be a full-time director who shall have no other major inpatient or service responsibility.

The Director of Ambulatory Care shall be a physician who is board-certified or qualified in internal medicine, general surgery, pediatrics, preventive medicine or public health.

DROP-IN CLINIC

The hospital will organize as part of its medical services a Drop-in Clinnic whose function it will be to care for those patients who come to the clinics without appointments. The function of the clinic will be to deal with the symptomatic relief of the presenting problem and shall be a referral source to other clinics.

EVENING CLINIC

The hospital shall establish an Evening Clinic which minimally will provide for the treatment in general medicine and in pediatrics. Said clinic to be open between the hours of 6 and 9 P.M.

NON-AVAILABILITY OF SERVICE

For services not available at the hospital, arrangements will be made and procedures established for referral to other health facilities providing the specific care needed.

CLINIC SCHEDULES

Clinic schedules will be available and conspicuously posted. They will be available in English as well as any other predominant languages representing those people making use of clinic services.

NUTRITION

The hospital will make available to the outpatient department the services of a nutritionist who will be available for consultation during regular clinic hours.

PREVENTIVE CARE

The outpatient department will provide preventive care in areas such as but not limited to venereal disease, well-baby, tuberculosis, etc.

SERVICES TO BE OFFERED

All basic medical services will be offered in the outpatient department including but not limited to medicine, Ob-Gyn, pediatrics, surgery and family planning.

STAFF TRAINING

The hospital will cause to have established an inservice education program for all levels of outpatient department staff, emphasizing those areas which will make them more professionally competent as well as giving them insight into human relationships and make them better equipped to deal with people on a more human level.

AUDITS

The Director of Ambulatory Care will cause to have established a system of outpatient department charts on a regular basis. Said audit to include the quality of medical care being offered.

UTILIZATION

The Director of Ambulatory Care will cause to have established a utilization review committee which will have as its responsibility reviewing and making recommendations relative to the utilization of all aspects of the outpatient department.

FOLLOW-UP CARE

A formal procedure will be established to follow up patients who have broken appointments. Provisions in the procedure will provide for both verbal and written reminders to patients for the next appointment.

STRUCTURE OF CARE

New patients shall insofar as medically indicated be referred first to the general medical and pediatric clinics for basic evaluation and screening. Subspecialty clinics shall be used only for consultation and for the management of those patients whose condition requires continuing subspecialty supervision.

Routine laboratory and X-ray procedures shall be made available on the day of patient's visit and insofar as possible shall not necessitate a return visit on another day purely for laboratory and X-ray procedures.

Summary Schedules D and E
of Ambulatory Care Program Contract, 1974

A publication of the Community Health Institute of New York City (M. F. McCann, *The Ambulatory Care Program: A Manual for Consumers*, New York: Community Health Institute, 1974) has neatly summarized these Schedules.

Highlights of Schedule D, the Outpatient Department Guidelines, are:

Comprehensive health care: Preventive health services should be provided, as well as diagnosis, treatment, and rehabilitation. New patients should be referred for a general medical or pediatric evaluation, and all patients who use the hospital as their primary source of medical care should have an annual complete physical examination. . . .

Continuity of care: Regular patients in the clinics should be seen by the same physician and nurses at each clinic visit. . . .

The hospital should provide the following services: medicine, pediatrics, surgery, obstetrics and gynecology, prenatal care. . . . General medical and general pediatric clinics should each have at least one session every day, Monday through Friday.

Services should be provided at hours most convenient to the patient, with the committee involved in deciding what those hours should be.

Regularly scheduled clinics should operate on an appointment basis only, but there should be a plan for caring for patients who come to the clinic without an appointment. There should be no more than a two-week wait for an appointment for a new patient. Thirty minutes should be allowed for a complete history and physical examination for a new patient. No more than five patients per hour per physician should be scheduled for re-visits. . . .

Clinic facilities should provide privacy for the patient during consultation, examination, and treatment.

A patient has the right to know the name of his physician, the nature and seriousness of his medical condition, and the treatment being provided for this condition.

The hospital should establish formal patient grievance procedures in consultation with the committee. . . .

Social workers should always be available in the general medical, general pediatric, pre-natal, abortion, and family planning clinics. . . .

A system which incorporates each patient's outpatient, inpatient, and emergency room charts into one record (a unit record system) should be established.

There should be a Director of Ambulatory Care who is the full-time director, with no other responsibilities. He should have sufficient authority and staff to carry out his responsibilities. All staff members shall be ultimately responsible to him for their work in the ambulatory care services. . . .

Schedule E includes the following standards:

The emergency room should be viewed as part of the total hospital services, with patients referred to the outpatient department or inpatient services if continued care is needed or desired.

At least one physician of resident level or higher and one registered nurse should be present in the emergency room seven days a week, twenty-four hours a day.

A professional staff person should be assigned to determine the seriousness of patients' problems and the order in which they will be treated. (This is known as a triage system.) . . . .

Lab and X-ray services should be available for immediate use at all times. . . .

A subcommittee of the hospital's audit committee should be established to review outpatient department and emergency room records to determine the quality and comprehensiveness of care . . .

All laboratory and X-ray reports for ambulatory services should be reviewed by a professional person within twenty-four hours of the completion of the test. . . .

Hospitals that do not have holding areas (where patients can remain for a period of time under observation before they are sent home or referred to the inpatient service) should establish them.

These standards are comprehensive and inclusive. One is continually impressed with the stress given in them to the quality of patient care.

Ambulatory Care Program:
Prototypical Case History/Evaluation Reports

From A. Schwarz, et al., *Evaluating Ambulatory Care in New York City*, New York: Department of Health, June, 1973, process:

The following material will present two examples which depict a cross-section of 26 hospitals which fall roughly into two categories: the large voluntary teaching hospital which is located such that it is eligible for Ghetto Medicine Program participation, and the small voluntary hospital, which is located in a ghetto area and which has lost or is losing all of its private patients and is forced, in order to survive, to become a "community hospital" in the fullest sense of the term.

The large voluntary teaching hospital generally is staffed with well-trained specialists, has a large number of subspecialty clinics, uses up-to-date techniques and modern laboratory equipment, has a large patient volume, is known for high quality in-patient service and, as a result of all of this, has a large operating budget and a high cost of operation.

What has the evaluation of ambulatory services to offer to an institution with so many recommendations? . . . How does the Bureau's philosophy of comprehensive, continuous, family-centered care rub up against a teaching hospital's philosophy?

To get an answer to these questions, consider what the site visit team finds upon its visit to a typical large, voluntary teaching hospital:

—The screening clinic is bulging at the seams and the medical and subspecialty clinics have a much more comfortable load of patients.

—There is a long wait (often 4 to 6 weeks) before a patient can be seen in the general medical clinic.

—Patients are sent to subspecialty clinics directly, from screening clinics and Emergency Room, without a complete work-up.

—The only clinic to which patients may "drop in" is the screening clinic. All other clinics operate strictly by appointment, with referrals made for an appointment from screening, Emergency Room, other clinics and inpatient service.

—The appointment books for several clinics have numerous blocks of time x'd out, or say no more than 6 patients.

—Many inpatients are wheeled from the floors into the subspecialty clinics.

—Nurses are filling out appointment slips and retrieving charts.

—The social workers in Outpatient Departments rotate through the clinics from the inpatient social service department.

—Chart review reveals a "ping-ponging" of patients between subspecialty clinics, with an occasional visit to screening clinic for treatment of an episodic illness. There are few nurses' notes.

—A consumer reports that she was sent from clinic to clinic until finally an oral surgeon to whom she was referred for a tooth extraction discovered that she had diabetes.

—Appointments to general clinics are made on a block-of-time basis to no particular physician, i.e., to medical clinic at 11:00 A.M.

—The broken appointment rate in several subspecialty clinics is rather high.

—Broken appointments for X-ray and laboratory work are not followed.

—X-ray and lab test results are not sent to the ordering physician or clinic; they are sent directly to the medical records room.

These disconnected and apparently unimportant pieces of information tell a large portion of the story of the health care delivery system at our hypothetical teaching hospital. . . .

In the site visit report, the chairman of the site-visit team will phrase the conclusions which tell the story of the health care delivery system of the hospital in such a way as to make the following points:

(1) The general clinics are not in fact available to many patients who might wish to use the hospital as their primary source of health care. They are forced to return to screening clinic or emergency room in order to get episodic care. They are sent from clinic to clinic with no one person having responsibility to coordinate the care they receive.

(2) Both the general and subspecialty clinics are wasteful of physician resources because they are not being utilized.

(3) Despite stable physician staffing patterns in the general clinics, continuity is not guaranteed.

(4) No method is set up to alert clinics that the patient did not keep an appointment for lab or X-ray procedure. Thus the patient may make a clinic visit wasteful of his time or of the doctor's.

(5) Care is disease-oriented rather than patient oriented.

(6) The Outpatient Department is not treated as an equal partner of the inpatient services.

(7) The Nurses are not performing nursing functions.

The recommendations of the site-visit team would be intended to deal with these problems. . . .

The second typical hospital is a small voluntary hospital located in the center of one of the large ghettos of New York City. It may still have some ties to a religious denomination; at one time it was a place where many of that denomination received their hospital care. Then, it was staffed by private physicians who would admit patients from all over the City. The Clinic and Emergency Room had small patient loads. The Clinic was largely for charity cases and the doctors volunteered to spend time there. Other clinic personnel were rotated through the Clinic—the less pleasant place to work—some troublesome physicians and nurses may even have been sent into exile there.

The Emergency room, like the Clinic area, has been expanded by carving out areas in the basement of the hospital; it has one small waiting room and a small examining/treatment room tucked away in some corner of the basement or ground floor, obviously suitable for ambulance cases only, but used for seeing 30,000 visits per year.

Within the last five years, the hospital has realized that it can no longer be the kind of hospital it once was. Its private patients no longer come and its voluntary physicians visit the hospital only occasionally. It is the only medical facility in an area of high medical need, and ambulatory visits has quadrupled in five years. Plans are being laid for a new hospital plant in the area, a real community hospital. But with all the delays, this will not be ready for at least five more years.

Staff attitudes keep this a voluntary hospital of 30 years ago. In fact, it is a primary physician, one might say *the* primary physician for the whole community around it. What is our same site visit team likely to observe in this hospital?

—Patients must make all appointments themselves: for return clinic visits, and for lab and X-ray, even routine work.

—The physical plant is run down, badly in need of paint and even basic maintenance.

—There is a huge language problem. Many of the patients cannot understand the physicians, and vice-versa.

—There is no unit record system. Separate records are kept in the OPD, and even abstracts of inpatients stays are not included in them.

—Patients come to the hospital clinic before the OPD doors are opened and may wait as long as 3-4 hours before they see a physician.

—Charts for clinic patients are not pulled in advance.

—The ER is for all practical purposes closed while the intern who is on duty is having his lunch and dinner.

—Triage is done by the registration clerk.

—Patients are being seen repeatedly in the ER. There is no system for making a follow-up appointment in clinic for an episode of illness.

—After the hospital pharmacy closes at 9 P.M. (2 P.M. on weekends), ER patients must have insurance or be able to pay the $10 emergency room fee plus lab and X-ray costs.

—Some effort is being made, informally, to assign patients to the same doctor on successive clinic visits. This takes the form of giving the patient an appointment on the day when the M.D. will be in clinic and then leaving it to the nurse to see that the patient sees that doctor.

—Appointments are given to sessions of the clinic; i.e., patients are given an appointment to Medical Clinic and are told to report at 8:30 A.M. Service is on a first-come, first-served basis.

—The attending physicians report late to Clinic, leave early, and see only three or four patients each session. The majority of the patients are seen by residents who must frequently stay beyond their session times. . . .

The recommendations which the Bureau will make to this hospital are:

(1) To clean up and paint the OPD and ER areas.

(2) To institute a unit record system.

(3) To develop a system of assigning each patient to a particular physician or nurse who will coordinate that patient's total care.

(4) To institute an appointment system which spreads the patient load over the sessions, say by giving appointments for 8:30, 9:30, 10:30, etc.

(5) To appoint patients to a specific physician.

(6) To institute a screening clinic to relieve the load on the ER, to provide an entry point into the Clinic system and to handle some of the drop-in patients.

(7) To disperse pre-packaged prescriptions through the ER when the hospital pharmacy is not open.

(8) To develop a triage system in the ER.

(9) To arrange physician coverage for ER when intern is having lunch and dinner.

(10) To develop a centralized appointment system where patient

can be given all necessary appointments (clinic, lab, and X-ray) at the same desk.

(11) To initiate a system whereby clinic patients would receive routine lab and X-ray tests not requiring special preparation on the same day as their present clinic visit.

(12) To consider amalgamating subspecialty clinics with the general clinics.

(13) To develop a system of improving the attending physician's attendance at clinics.

(14) To develop a means of following ER patients in the Clinics after their first visit to the ER.

All too conclusively the Hospitals in the Ghetto Medicine Program offer stopgap, episodic care to too many persons in situations where comprehensive ambulatory care is called for both medically and in terms of the Ghetto Medicine Contract.

Ghetto Medicine as it now stands is based on the premise that reorganization of the health system in New York City must start at the core of the voluntary sector, where the most power lies. A reorganization in this core is urgently needed. Ghetto Medicine can bring it about only through a commitment to maximum pressure for comprehensive care and stringent enforcement of the mandates in the Ghetto Medicine Contract and Guidelines.

APPENDIX 12

Suffolk County Department of Health Services, Division of Patient Care Services: Guidelines, Community Advisory Board

I. PURPOSE

To advise the Comissioner of Health Services, charged with the general supervision and control over the operations of Health Centers, and the Back-up hospital regarding services.

A. To enhance Health Center services through the involvement of the Hospital and the Department of Health Services with its community.

B. To insure that Health Center services are meeting the health needs of the community and that personalized and dignified care is being rendered.

C. To make recommendations aimed towards increasing sensitivity of the Health Center administration to its constituency, the people it serves.

D. Involvement in the planning, developing, and evaluation of the services being rendered.

E. To facilitate appropriate community utilization of available services by assisting in the dissemination of information in the community about these services and acting as health advocates; reports of such activities will be made to the Joint Administrative Committee.

II. SCOPE OF PARTICIPATION

The Community Advisory Board shall advise and consult with the Commissioner and the Hospital on the following, as related to Health Center services:

A. Physical plant standards

B. Maintenance of facilities

C. Procedures for fee collection

D. Staffing patterns

E. Establishment of health priorities

F. Hours of service

G. Review and follow-up of patient grievances

III. IMPLEMENTATION

A. The Commissioner of Health Services will appoint Community Advisory Board members to a term of one year; appointments will be

171

made with the assistance of an Ad Hoc Committee of active community groups and individuals.

    1. A short biographical sketch should be submitted for each candidate.

    B. The Community Advisory Board shall have a membership numbering at least seven; the membership shall have a majority of at least 51% consumers, i.e., active users of services. It will be the responsibility of the Community Advisory Board to meet and maintain this standard.

    C. Representative of the Department of Health Services, Hospital Administration, and Health Center Administration shall serve as ex-officio members; extension of voting privileges to ex-officio members shall be determined by each Community Advisory Board.

    D. The Community Advisory Board shall have an annual membership drive and election of officers. It shall develop its own by-laws in consonance with these guidelines and subject to the review of back-up hospital and approval of the Commissioner.

    E. The Community Advisory Board shall appoint several subcommittees for the purpose of carrying out board work functions. Examples of such subcommittees are: Program and Budget; Membership; Legislative; Education; Space; Personnel, etc.

    F. Meetings should be at least six times annually, and shall have a quorum of members present to constitute an official meeting. Open meetings shall be held annually.

    1. Should be scheduled at least two weeks in advance to give all participants sufficient notice.

    2. Questions of procedure shall be determined according to Robert's Rules of Order.

    3. Should be time-limited.

    4. Minutes shall be regularly submitted to the Commissioner.

    G. The Community Advisory Board will be given the opportunity to review proposed major program changes in advance of their adoption.

    H. The Community Advisory Board shall have the right to have all public reports and documents pertaining to the Health Center made available to them, i.e., annual budget requests and allocations, periodic statistical reports, etc.; and the obligation to use these in a responsible manner.

    K. The Community Advisory Board shall advise in the personnel selection process in the following way:

    1. The Community Advisory Board shall make recommendations as to the characteristics deemed important in personnel.

    2. The Community Advisory Board will appoint two members to

advise in the selection process for the Medical Director, Administrator, and Nursing Supervisor.

    a. Candidates will first be screened by the Administration for acceptability.

    b. Community Advisory Board representatives will advise on acceptability.

    c. Supporting data should be forwarded for candidates deemed not acceptable. Can be brief, but as specific as possible.

L. Each Health Center shall have a Joint Administrative Committee. This Committee shall have one representative each from the Department of Health Services, the Back-up Hospital, and the Health Center, and the Community Advisory Board. Attendance at Committee Meetings will not exceed two members from each of the above-listed groups, except with prior notice and approval of the Committee. Where voting is required, one vote each will be accorded the Hospital, the Community Board, and the Department of Health Services.

M. Each Community Advisory Board shall have space made available to them on Health Center premises to carry out its functions, amongst which will be the role of patient advocacy; i.e., a patient with a grievance, having exhausted without satisfaction his right to consult with Health Center personnel, will be free to request the intervention of the Community Advisory Board.

N. A designated sum of money shall be budgeted for reimbursement of board members for such miscellaneous expenses as stationery, stamps, printing, recording tapes, etc.